11/4

D0953456

MAYO CLINIC

Going Gluten FREE

Published by Time Home Entertainment Inc.
1271 Avenue of the Americas
New York, NY 10020

ISBN-10: 0-8487-4388-1
ISBN-13: 978-0-8487-4388-8

Library of Congress Control Number: 2014946271

Mayo Clinic Going Gluten-Free is intended to supplement the advice of your personal physician, whom you should consult regarding individual medical conditions. MAYO, MAYO CLINIC, and the Mayo triple-shield logo are marks of Mayo Foundation for Medical Education and Research.

We welcome your comments and suggestions about Time Home Entertainment books. Please write to Time Home Entertainment books, Attention: Book Editors, P.O. Box 11016, Des Moines, IA 50336-1016.

If you would like to order any of our hardcover Collector's Edition books, please call us at 800-327-6388, Monday through Friday, 7 a.m. to 8 p.m., or Saturday, 7 a.m. to 6 p.m., Central time.

For bulk sales to employers, member groups and health-related companies, contact Mayo Clinic, 200 First St. SW, Rochester, MN 55905, or send an email to the following address: SpecialSalesMayoBooks@Mayo.edu.

We do not endorse any company or product.

Printed in the United States of America

PHOTO CREDITS

There is no correlation between the individuals portrayed and the conditions or subjects discussed.

CREDIT: © MAYO FOUNDATION FOR MEDICAL EDUCATION AND RESEARCH (MFMER) – NAME: 78781383.PSD/CHAPTER 2/CREDIT: © THINKSTOCK – NAME: 179298912.PSD/CHAPTER 4/CREDIT: © THINKSTOCK – NAME: 112796301.PSD/CHAPTER 4/CREDIT: © THINKSTOCK – NAME: 470047657.PSD/CHAPTER 4/CREDIT: © THINKSTOCK – NAME: 491451015.PSD/CHAPTER 4/CREDIT: © THINKSTOCK – NAME: 179695098.PSD/CHAPTER 5/CREDIT: © THINKSTOCK – NAME: 178180556.PSD/CHAPTER 6/CREDIT: © THINKSTOCK – NAME: 488667731.PSD/CHAPTER 6/CREDIT: © THINKSTOCK – NAME: 56570208.PSD/CHAPTER 7/CREDIT: © THINKSTOCK – NAME: 122413055-COUPLERUNNING.PSD/CHAPTER 9/CREDIT: © THINKSTOCK – NAME: 154127632.PSD/CHAPTER 10/CREDIT: © THINKSTOCK – NAME: 493631953.PSD/CHAPTER 11/CREDIT: © THINKSTOCK – NAME: 78459195.PSD/CHAPTER 11/CREDIT: © THINKSTOCK – NAME: AA052181_20.PSD/CHAPTER 11/CREDIT: © THINKSTOCK – NAME: 156970153.PSD/CHAPTER 12/CREDIT: © THINKSTOCK – NAME: 156970153.PSD/CHAPTER 12/CREDIT: © THINKSTOCK – NAME: 164545244.PSD/CHAPTER 12/CREDIT: © THINKSTOCK – NAME: 164545244.PSD/CHAPTER 12/CREDIT: © THINKSTOCK – NAME: 164542881.PSD/CHAPTER 12/CREDIT: © THINKSTOCK – NAME: 156970153.PSD/CHAPTER 12/CREDIT: © THINKSTOCK – NAME: 453531537.PSD/CHAPTER 12/CREDIT: © THINKSTOCK – NAME: 178384095.PSD/CHAPTER 12/CREDIT: © THINKSTOCK – NAME: 179245502.JPG/CHAPTER 12/CREDIT: © THINKSTOCK – NAME: 452240637.JPG/CHAPTER 12/CREDIT: © THINKSTOCK – NAME: 469951011.JPG/CHAPTER 12/CREDIT: © THINKSTOCK – NAME: 177109425.JPG/CHAPTER 12/CREDIT: © THINKSTOCK – NAME: 452167741.JPG/CHAPTER 12/CREDIT: © THINKSTOCK – NAME: 160581649.JPG/CHAPTER 12/CREDIT: © THINKSTOCK – NAME: 184714755.JPG/CHAPTER 12/CREDIT: © THINKSTOCK – NAME: 459953661.JPG/CHAPTER 12/CREDIT: © THINKSTOCK – NAME: 158478547.PSD/CHAPTER 13/CREDIT: © THINKSTOCK – NAME: 103966019.PSD/CHAPTER 14/CREDIT: © THINKSTOCK – NAME: 92890195.PSD/CHAPTER 14/CREDIT: © THINKSTOCK – NAME: 470794829.PSD/CHAPTER 15/CREDIT: © THINKSTOCK – NAME: 178622548.PSD/CHAPTER 15/CREDIT: © THINKSTOCK – NAME: 467371507.PSD/CHAPTER 15/CREDIT: © THINKSTOCK – NAME: 177305184.PSD/CHAPTER 15/CREDIT: © THINKSTOCK – NAME: 106534008.PSD/CHAPTER 15/CREDIT: © THINKSTOCK – NAME: 460843611.PSD/CHAPTER 15/CREDIT: © THINKSTOCK – NAME: 200464182-001.PSD/CHAPTER 16/CREDIT: © THINKSTOCK – NAME: 166736459.PSD/CHAPTER 16/CREDIT: © THINKSTOCK – NAME: 77832666.PSD/CHAPTER 17/CREDIT: © THINKSTOCK – NAME: 56383069.PSD/CHAPTER 18/CREDIT: © THINKSTOCK – NAME: 153755289.PSD/CHAPTER 18/CREDIT: © THINKSTOCK –

MAYO CLINIC

Medical Editor
Joseph A. Murray, M.D.

Associate Medical Editor
Jacalyn A. See, L.D.

Managing Editor
Karen R. Wallevand

Contributors
Imad Absah, M.D.
Rachel A. H. Bartony
Alicia C. Bartz
Julie A. Buchholtz, L.D.
Manish J. Gandhi, M.D.
Kevin G. Kaufman
Vandana Nehra, M.D.
Jennifer K. Nelson, RDN, L.D.
Miguel A. Park, M.D.
John A. Schaffner, M.D.
Richard J. Seime, Ph.D., L.P.
Melissa R. Snyder, Ph.D.
Suzanne P. Sobotka
Maria I. Vazquez Roque, M.D.
Laura Hamilton Waxman

Editorial Director
Paula Marlow Limbeck

Product Manager
Christopher C. Frye

Art Director
Richard A. Resnick

Illustrators and Photographers
Joanna R. King
Malgorzata B. (Gosha) Weivoda

Research Librarians
Amanda K. Golden
Deirdre A. Herman

Proofreaders
Miranda M. Attlesey
Donna L. Hanson
Julie M. Maas

Indexer
Steve Rath

Administrative Assistant
Beverly J. Steele

TIME HOME ENTERTAINMENT INC.

President and Publisher
Jim Childs

Vice President and Associate Publisher
Margot Schupf

Vice President, Finance
Vandana Patel

Executive Director, Marketing Services
Carol Pittard

Publishing Director
Megan Pearlman

Associate General Counsel
Simone Procas

Senior Manager, Business Development & Partnerships
Nina Fleishman Reed

OXMOOR HOUSE

Editorial Director
Leah McLaughlin

Creative Director
Felicity Keane

Art Director
Christopher Rhoads

Executive Food Director
Grace Parisi

Managing Editor
Elizabeth Tyler Austin

Assistant Managing Editor
Jeanne de Lathouder

Special thanks to Greg A. Amason, Allyson Angle, Katherine Barnet, Jeremy Biloon, Susan Chodakiewicz, Rose Cirrincione, Jacqueline Fitzgerald, Christine Font, Jenna Goldberg, Hillary Hirsch, David Kahn, Mona Li, Amy Mangus, Amy Migliaccio, Nina Mistry, Dave Rozzelle, Ricardo Santiago, Adriana Tierno, Vanessa Wu

Cover design by Christopher Rhoads

My journey with celiac disease started in Galway in the West of Ireland, where celiac disease was remarkably common in the 1960s and '70s. My alma mater, the National University of Ireland in Galway, became a center for celiac disease research. As a medical student and intern, I regarded celiac disease as part of the medical landscape; it seemed to be as commonplace as hypertension or heart disease. It left me with the impression that celiac disease was far more common than perhaps was known at the time. My journey with celiac disease continued in Dublin, and I can vividly recall the last patient that I diagnosed before leaving Ireland to come to America. It was a young woman who had few, if any, gastrointestinal symptoms. I also recall my mentor telling me that this would likely be the last patient with celiac disease I would see because the disease was rare in the United States.

My move across the Atlantic wasn't to follow celiac disease but to pursue my interest in other gastrointestinal disorders. But in the Iowa cornfields, I discovered celiac disease. It's rare that a single patient can so influence a career, but at The University of Iowa I met a woman who broke the mold for how celiac disease was supposed to act. She was overweight not under-weight, had constipation not diarrhea, lost weight on a gluten-free diet and gained weight when she ate gluten.

Recognizing that the celiac disease I was seeing in the United States wasn't the celiac disease of Ireland piqued my interest, and I began to look for the disease outside of the usual places. With the advent of widespread endoscopy, which made it possible to see and biopsy the small intestine where celiac disease develops, my interest developed into a zeal, and before I left Iowa there were almost 100 new cases of celiac disease diagnosed in 1997.

My years in Iowa gave me a new appreciation for celiac disease. At this time, there was little information available for patients, little awareness of the disease among most physicians and the general population, virtually no commercially available gluten-free foods, no labeling standards, and few specialized gluten-free suppliers. Truth be told, the gluten-free foods provided by mostly mom and pop operations were not very tasty.

My move to Mayo Clinic in 1998 offered an opportunity to work in one of the very best medical centers dedicated to not only outstanding clinical care but also care provided in a highly organized fashion. It provided a platform to develop both a celiac disease clinic and a multiple site program that today includes Rochester, Minnesota; Jacksonville, Florida; and Phoenix/Scottsdale Arizona. Mayo's program includes one of the largest celiac laboratories. The opportunity to work with colleagues dedicated to advancing the science of celiac disease while at the same time recognizing the needs of our patients has been exciting and rewarding.

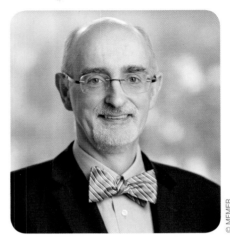

Joseph A. Murray, M.D.
Medical editor

There's much we have learned and much still to be learned in this rapidly changing field. Gluten has become front and center in the public eye and is garnering greater medical, governmental and industry interest. Celiac disease has emerged from the shadows. Questions of how to find it, how to cure it, and, particularly, how to prevent it are key challenges for the next two decades.

This book is a culmination of not only my two decades studying and treating celiac disease but also the endeavors, talents and expertise of many of the Mayo Clinic team who work in the celiac field. I hope that you find the book informative and helpful for whatever stage of contemplation, diagnosis, treatment or follow-up you're at, be it celiac disease or another gluten- or wheat-related disorder.

I am very grateful to the patients, colleagues, friends and especially my wife Imelda who have made this book possible.

CONTENTS

The gluten story

Gluten — or more specifically, our desire to avoid it — is taking the health food market by storm. The words *gluten-free* are everywhere — the grocery store, the bakery, on restaurant menus and in bookstores. Many people seem to be going to great lengths to rid gluten from their diets. So what is it about gluten that has so many people wanting it off their plates?

If you're holding this book you may already know a little about gluten and want to learn more. Or maybe you don't know a thing about it, but you're curious. You might wonder if the discomfort you sometimes feel after eating could be related to gluten. You'd like to know if eating less gluten will make you healthier. Perhaps you're debating if your entire family might be better off following a gluten-free diet.

The gluten story is complex. Regardless of whether you need to avoid gluten or you simply want to, in this book we'll help you sort out fact from fiction — what we know about gluten, what we don't, and what doctors and researchers speculate could be going on.

The first section of the book is devoted to celiac disease, an illness caused by eating gluten. You'll learn how to recognize symptoms, how the disease is diagnosed, and how to manage a gluten-free lifestyle. This is followed by a discussion of other gluten- and wheat-related disorders with similar signs and symptoms that may or may not be related to eating gluten. You'll learn about non-celiac gluten sensitivity, which has received a lot of press lately.

The last part of the book is a practical guide to the ins and outs of gluten-free living. Whether you need to or want to avoid gluten, this section is your ticket to discovering new ways of eating well to help you feel your best. You'll learn the basics of a gluten-free diet, how to stock your kitchen, make wise choices when eating out and even help a child transition to a gluten-free diet.

But first things first: What is gluten anyway? And why is it such a problem for a growing number of people?

What is gluten?

If you've ever mixed flour with water, you know that within seconds you're likely to have a kind of sticky, spongy mess on your hands. Given the right ratios and some salt, leavening and fat, along with a few minutes of kneading, you soon have a ball of smooth, elastic dough on your hands.

Gluten — a protein composite found in the heart of the grassy grains wheat, barley and rye — is what transforms the dry and wet ingredients into the stretchy stuff in front of you. Normally, these proteins serve as storage houses for nutrients that support seed germination and growth. But when the proteins are mixed with liquid, they create an elastic matrix that's able to expand and help a food maintain its intended shape. When combined with a leavening such as yeast, the gluten matrix captures bubbles of carbon dioxide given off by the yeast's fermentation and rises to produce the texture and shape of, say a chewy baguette or a tall sandwich loaf.

Wheat and wheat variants and byproducts, including durum, bulgur, semolina, spelt and couscous, are the most well-known sources of gluten. But other grains also contain gluten, including barley and rye. In modern society, foods made with wheat are practically everywhere. Because of their ability to lend elasticity and airiness, gluten-rich wheat flour or purified gluten (vital gluten) are added to almost all baked products. Wheat is also a main ingredient in most pastas and cereals. Malt, made from barley, also contains gluten. Malt is central to the making of beer and some vinegars.

Gluten also is used as a stabilizer, flavor enhancer or thickening agent in other food products such as soy sauce, soups, salad dressings and even ice cream. And it's in products you wouldn't expect. Not obvious yet potential sources of gluten include vitamins, medications, communion wafers and even modeling clay.

Why gluten is a problem

In ancient times, wheat grew wild. Archaeological evidence from the Fertile Crescent along the Tigris and Euphrates rivers in the Middle East suggests that humans ground up wheat to make food but only what they were able to collect in the wild. Gradually, however, humans began to save grain seeds and plant them in specific spots, thus beginning the cultivation of wheat as a crop. This domestication of wheat — estimated to have occurred about 10,000 years ago — helped create more reliable and accessible sources of food, allowing humans to move from being hunters and gatherers to living in a more stable, agricultural society. Today, wheat is everywhere. And the gluten found in wheat has become a common ingredient in many foods because it helps bread and other foods maintain their shape and texture. But as wheat, as well as barley and rye, have evolved and become more abundant, so have issues related to their consumption.

The problem is, gluten is often poorly digested. While moving through your small intestine, components of gluten are absorbed whole into the lining of the small intestine. There, the components are broken down by certain enzymes. This process in itself isn't bad, but for reasons that aren't clear, for some people it's a recipe for trouble, causing them more harm than good. What researchers have found is that for people who carry a particular genetic code, gluten can trigger a harmful reaction in the intestine. This intestinal reaction is the hallmark of celiac disease.

If you have celiac disease and you eat something that contains gluten, the immune reaction that results inflames and swells the inner lining of your small intestine. The inflammation and swelling may cause problems with digestion and absorption, producing gastrointestinal symptoms such as diarrhea and abdominal cramps. But more significantly, continued exposure to gluten can damage your small intestine to the point where it's unable to absorb nutrients, leaving you without essential vitamins and minerals important to your health. Ultimately, this can lead to serious illness. The only way to treat celiac disease is by completely eliminating gluten from your diet.

Aside from celiac disease, wheat can cause other problems. A small number of people are allergic to one or more of the various proteins found in wheat. If a person with a wheat allergy eats wheat or even inhales wheat flour, he or she may have an allergic reaction with symptoms such as a skin rash, lip swelling, wheezing or difficulty breathing, abdominal pain, and diarrhea. Some may even experience a life-threatening reaction called anaphylaxis.

Wheat allergy and celiac disease are sometimes confused, but the two are very different conditions. What is similar about them, though, and what often ties them together, is that to avoid illness, it's critical to avoid wheat.

Most recently, the notion has surfaced that some people may have a condition called non-celiac gluten sensitivity. It's not the same as celiac disease, but it may produce similar symptoms, such as abdominal discomfort and feelings of tiredness. What's interesting is that in this case public interest is driving the science. Many people who haven't been diagnosed with celiac disease are opting to live gluten-free in an effort to relieve their symptoms, claiming they feel better when they eliminate gluten from their diets. As a result, researchers are investigating whether there may be a gluten disorder — a type of sensitivity — that's a milder form of celiac disease, a condition sometimes referred to as "celiac-lite."

Non-celiac gluten sensitivity is tricky to identify, though. There are no diagnostic tests for it, and there are more questions about this condition than there are answers. In fact, doctors still aren't certain if gluten is responsible for symptoms of the disorder or if it might be another component of grain.

Gluten- and wheat-related disorders are nothing new. They've been around for thousands of years, but interest in them has increased considerably just in the past decade. More people appear to be developing celiac disease than ever before — it's clearly a disease on the rise. And the notion that celiac disease or even non-celiac gluten sensitivity may be the cause of a host of common ailments, ranging from chronic abdominal pain to fatigue to dementia, has captured the public imagination. In the meantime, scientists are ramping up efforts to try to figure out what exactly is going on.

The gluten-free movement

In light of all the attention being given to gluten, it's not surprising that the idea of a gluten-free lifestyle has quickly become mainstream. Marketing surveys suggest many Americans are trying to cut down on gluten or avoid it entirely. This may be bolstered, in part, by a few best-selling authors who claim that to lose weight you have to "lose the wheat," or that grains, gluten and carbohydrates are a hazard to brain and heart health. Millions of Americans have decided to pursue a gluten-free diet, often without seeking medical advice first. And the amount of money being spent on gluten-free products is well into the billions of dollars annually, with sales expected to increase.

The food industry, meanwhile, is happy to comply. Labeling a product gluten-free can increase its appeal to a fairly broad range of consumers. Major supermarket chains have joined the ranks of health food stores and now dedicate whole aisles to gluten-free foods. Some of the big cereal companies are even muscling in on the action, introducing gluten-free cereals. Gluten-free bakeries are popping up in trendy neighborhoods, and gluten-free items are featured prominently on an increasing number of restaurant menus.

Health and wellness are popular themes in American life, and many Americans are willing, if not anxious, to try new products or programs they think might help them live and feel better. As with any diet, however, eliminating a single component doesn't automatically make you healthier. Increasing your consumption of fruits and vegetables, which are naturally gluten-free, is likely to improve your health, especially if you're eating them in place of pizza and doughnuts. But if you're swapping gluten-free cookies for wheat-based crackers, and eating more of the cookies than you did the crackers, you may not be doing your health much of a favor. In addition, an unbalanced gluten-free diet can lead to deficiencies in a number of vitamins and minerals commonly used in fortified wheat and wheat-based products.

Also keep in mind that if you begin a gluten-free diet before you have a chance to be evaluated by your doctor, you may not be able to find out if you have celiac disease. To get an accurate diagnosis, you need to be eating food containing gluten when tests for the disease are performed.

Fortunately, for people who need to avoid gluten for medical reasons, and even for those who just want to, many more gluten-free foods are now available, and eating out is actually within the realm of possibility in most locations. Increased awareness of gluten-related disorders has increased support for gluten-free products. Remember, though, that anyone can follow a gluten-free lifestyle. The key is to do it right — to make sure you're not only cutting out all gluten and protecting your physical health, but you're adopting an eating plan that you can truly live with.

That's what this book is about — how to go gluten-free safely and enjoy it!

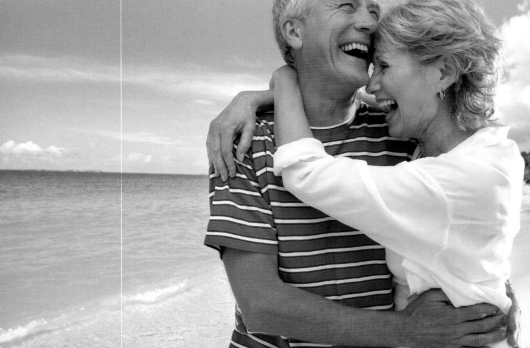

LISA'S STORY

I was in my early 20s when I started having symptoms. After certain meals I would feel very nauseated. I sensed a burning at the top of my stomach, followed by tightness and bloating. After the food was through my system, I would feel normal again.

I knew something wasn't right, so I went to a doctor who diagnosed me with irritable bowel syndrome. I never thought that's what I had, and I knew the sickness I felt was linked to eating specific foods.

Over the next few years, I also started getting headaches with the nausea. At age 39, I began noticing that my left hand and foot felt weak and a little bit numb. I was sent to a neurologist who diagnosed me with a nerve condition and prescribed medication that made me tired and sick. When the numbness started progressing to my other foot and hand, I saw a new doctor who took me off the medication and tested me for multiple sclerosis, lupus, hepatitis C and a number of other things. Two years later, I ended up with a diagnosis of idiopathic neuropathy, the medical term for unexplained nerve inflammation. I was feeling worse and experiencing headaches almost daily.

I was used to exercising over my lunch hour, but I had to stop. My joints hurt, my back hurt, my neck hurt, and I also had a great deal of pain from the neuropathy in my feet. I was 42 years old and felt like I was 90.

Eventually, I was referred to Mayo Clinic. It was a last ditch effort to figure out what was wrong with me. And, thankfully, I got my answer. Blood tests for celiac disease came back positive. The results were confirmed by a biopsy of my upper intestine, which showed significant intestinal damage. The doctor said that under a microscope my intestine looked like a flat tile floor.

So there it was. Finally! It was almost too good to believe.

I learned that by changing my diet I could cure my body. The first week eating gluten-free was overwhelming. We live in a small town, and we don't have stores with lots of gluten-free food. Eventually, I was connected with a doctor at our local hospital who has celiac disease. He told me where to buy gluten-free food and which local restaurants have gluten-free items on the menu. I'm trying to eat healthier whole foods, and I'm glad to be eliminating processed foods from my diet. In just a month, my headaches have gone away, I feel like I have more energy, and my stomach feels good.

Both of our sons tested negative for celiac disease. However, they both have similar stomach problems when they eat. I know they can test positive when they're older, so we'll continue to monitor them.

My family has been great through the entire ordeal. I think they're as relieved as I am to finally have it all figured out.

Celiac Disease

CHAPTER ONE

Understanding celiac disease

It wasn't that long ago that few people had even heard of celiac disease. It's still not a common illness, especially when you compare it with conditions such as heart disease or cancer. But awareness of celiac disease is increasing, and a major reason why is because the disease is growing in numbers. At the same time, researchers are learning more about the disease — how it evolves and how it acts. For years, doctors associated celiac disease with underweight individuals who frequently complained of belly pain and diarrhea. It's now clear that the disease can behave differently in different people, and you don't have to be skinny or even have digestive problems to have celiac disease.

Did you know ?

The number of people currently being told they have celiac disease is almost 20 times greater than the number of people diagnosed with the disease just 20 years ago. Once thought to occur only in children, celiac disease can affect people of any age, from infants to older adults. In fact, today the disease is more common in adults than in children — the average age at diagnosis is about 45.

Regardless of whether you've been diagnosed with celiac disease or you think you could be at risk, one of the first and most important steps you can take is to learn all you can about the illness. Knowing why it occurs, what it does to your body and how it's treated will help you understand why you feel the way you do and what you need to do to stay healthy. Managing celiac disease is pretty straightforward: it's all about diet. What's more complex is how the disease expresses itself. Many people live with celiac disease for years before finally learning what's wrong with them.

An immune system malfunction

So what exactly is celiac disease? It's an immune disorder. And what is that? It's a condition in which your own immune system is harming you. In the case of celiac disease, when you eat foods that contain gluten, your immune system responds to the gluten the same as it does a foreign invader — it tries to attack and destroy it. The trouble is, your small intestine pays the price. The constant attack on gluten irritates and inflames your small intestine, preventing the absorption of key nutrients. Eventually, this deprives your body of vital nourishment, leading to illnesses. In children, the disease can affect growth and development.

What causes your body to react this way? Similar to many immune disorders, it's thought to be an interplay between genetics and something in the environment. Oftentimes, neither the faulty genetic code nor the environmental trigger is known, leaving doctors and individuals with the disorder in the dark as to how it developed and how best to treat it. Fortunately, with celiac disease, a lot is known about the genes that make people susceptible to the illness and, of course, the primary environmental trigger is gluten.

To successfully treat celiac disease, it's crucial that you eliminate gluten. A gluten-free diet can help you feel better within a matter of weeks and over time cause healing of your small intestine.

Your digestive system

Much of the damage caused by celiac disease occurs where you can't see or sometimes even feel it — within your digestive system. When you eat food that contains gluten, your digestive system, particularly your small intestine, reacts abnormally. To understand how celiac disease affects your digestive system, it helps to understand what normally happens when you eat.

NORMAL DIGESTION When you eat, you nourish your body. However, for your body to absorb the nutrients from the food you consume, each bite must be broken down into smaller and smaller pieces until the nutrients are small enough to be absorbed into your bloodstream and carried to your tissues, muscles and various organs.

The first step occurs when you chew. Your teeth tear the food into smaller pieces while your tongue mixes the pieces with saliva, reducing the food to a mushy consistency. When you swallow, the food is propelled down the back part of your throat and into your esophagus, where wavelike muscle contractions (peristalsis) move the food into your stomach. Powerful muscles in your stomach churn food into even smaller pieces and mix them with gastric juices so that by the time food leaves the stomach and enters your small intestine it resembles more of a thick liquid.

Very little food is actually absorbed by your stomach. That job is mostly performed by your small intestine. The first part of the small intestine (duodenum) prepares the food for maximum absorption, along with the help of digestive juices from your liver, gallbladder and pancreas.

The next and largest part of your intestine (jejunum) is where the majority of absorption takes place. Here, additional enzymes further break down carbohydrates, proteins and fats, as well as vitamins and minerals, so that they can be absorbed through the intestinal lining and transferred into your bloodstream, from which they'll circulate to the rest of your body.

This absorption process relies heavily on millions of tiny hairlike projections called villi that line the intestine. Villi resemble the deep pile of a plush carpet on a microscopic scale. Their job is to capture nutrients and move them into the intestinal lining. The real work of absorption is done by tiny cells located on the surface of the villi. They provide a large working surface equal in size to about two tennis courts.

The last part of your small intestine (ileum) absorbs any remaining nutrients and much of the water in the small intestine. The ileum is responsible for passage of what's left of the food you ate into the large intestine (colon). Here, the role of your digestive system changes. Now its job is to process the remaining waste, which consists mainly of water, fiber and unabsorbed food. The liquid is absorbed into the bloodstream, while the rest of the waste material moves through the colon and collects in the rectum until the next bowel movement.

CELIAC DISEASE Gluten is a protein found in wheat, barley and rye. When you ingest gluten, certain parts of the gluten molecule called gliadin peptides tend to resist being broken down by the digestive process. This happens with everyone, whether you have celiac disease or not.

Normally, your intestinal lining forms a tight barrier that keeps these kinds of large undigested molecules out. But with celiac disease, chemical

Digestive system

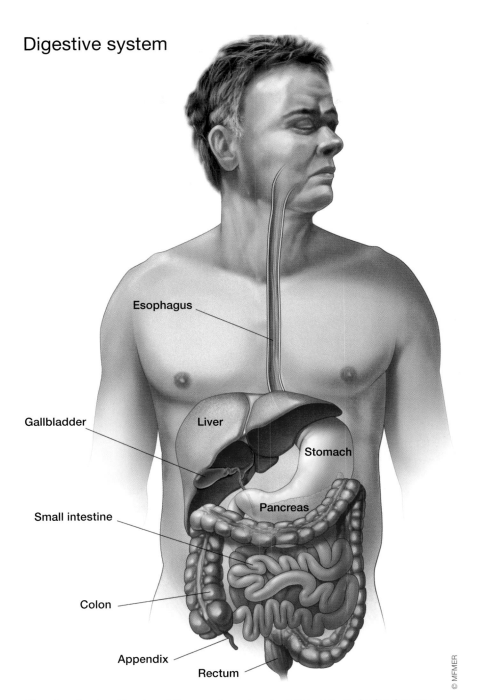

The digestive tract begins at the mouth and ends at the rectum. As food moves along the digestive tract, it's broken down into particles, vital nutrients are absorbed from the food particles, and remaining waste exits the rectum in the form of stool.

changes occur that alter the intestinal lining, allowing the peptides to filter through. Once past this barrier, a complex series of interactions occur at the cellular level that cause a showdown between the body's immune system and the gliadin peptides. The immune system treats the peptides as if they were harmful and consequently mounts an inflammatory attack against them.

When the immune system overreacts in this way, the small intestine becomes inflamed and the villi that line the small intestine are damaged. This damage eventually causes the inner surface of the small intestine to appear more like a tile floor than the plush carpet it's supposed to resemble. As a result, nutrients travel through the damaged intestine unabsorbed rather than being caught up by villi and processed into your bloodstream.

But not all of the small intestine is affected at once. The damage from celiac disease tends to occur in patches (see the opposite page). In most cases, villi in the duodenum and jejunum are damaged before those in the ileum. This means that when the upper portions of the small intestine are unable to function properly, the ileum will try to make up for them, digesting food and absorbing nutrients in a way that usually occurs upstream in the digestive tract.

In fact, the villi in the ileum often grow bigger to accommodate the changes. So even though your upper intestine may be damaged by celiac disease, your lower intestine may still be able to absorb enough nutrients so that you don't experience malabsorption. This adaptive nature of the ileum helps explain why many people with celiac disease don't have classic signs and symptoms of the disease, including malnourishment and weight loss.

An unhealthy recipe

Scientists know quite a bit about what ingredients are needed for celiac disease to develop. Research shows that when two, and sometimes three, factors are combined, it's a recipe for illness.

GENETICS Genetics plays an integral role in celiac disease. For a person to develop the disease — whether in early childhood or later in life — certain genes that make you susceptible to the condition almost always are present.

Scientists have discovered that specific genes belonging to the human leukocyte antigen (HLA) gene family that encode for molecules called HLA-DQ2 and HLA-DQ8 are crucial to the development of celiac disease. Almost all individuals with celiac disease carry the genetic markers that encode these genes. It's natural to think of these as "bad" genes. However, the HLA genes aren't actually abnormal genes or even harmful outside of their involvement in celiac disease. They've persisted through human development, probably because of some advantage they provided to those that carried them.

Celiac disease

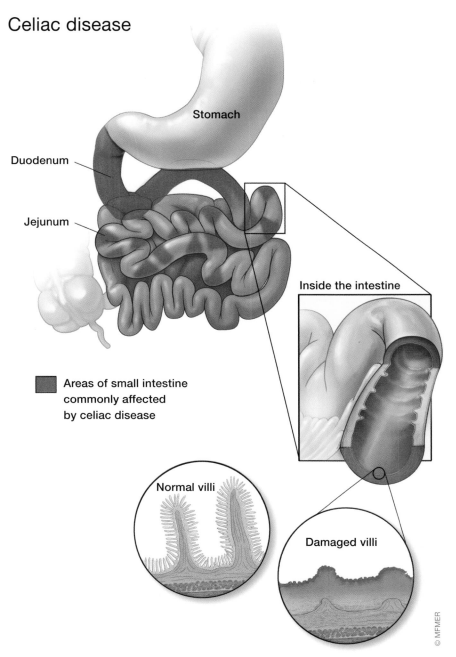

Stomach

Duodenum

Jejunum

Areas of small intestine commonly affected by celiac disease

Inside the intestine

Normal villi

Damaged villi

© MFMER

Nutrients in food are absorbed by hairlike projections in the small intestine called villi. Celiac disease damages villi, so they can't absorb nutrients. The first section of the small intestine (duodenum) is where most of the damage typically occurs, with patches of disease in the middle portion of the small intestine (jejunum).

The origins of celiac disease date back to the Greeks

Celiac disease, once more commonly known as celiac sprue, has actually been around for a long time — probably ever since wheat was introduced to the human diet. The earliest description of celiac disease is attributed to the Greek physician, Aretaeus. He coined the term *koiliakos* — after the Greek word *koelia* for abdomen — which translates to English as "celiac." Aretaeus described people who couldn't retain their food and passed it through "undigested."

In the late 1800s, English physician Samuel Jones Gee published a detailed description of celiac disease symptoms in children and suggested that treatment would most likely have to be through diet. For many years, celiac disease was thought to be an illness that primarily affected children from Northern Europe. When a child showed obvious signs and symptoms — mainly chronic diarrhea and malnutrition — and there was no other explanation for the symptoms, the child was diagnosed with celiac disease.

What caused the disease remained unknown until as recently as 1940, when gluten's central role was discovered. Dutch pediatrician Willem K. Dicke, who treated children with celiac symptoms, suspected that diet played a role, and he noticed during the bread shortages of World War II his young patients improved but relapsed when bread and cereal became readily available again. This prompted Dicke and a colleague to conduct studies on the children that confirmed wheat, barley and rye (and oats to a degree) were the culprits. Not long after, gluten was identified as the key protein responsible for the disease.

In the 1970s, blood tests were introduced that identified a particular set of antibodies signaling the body's immune reaction to gluten, and hence a marker for celiac disease that could easily be assessed. Doctors were also becoming aware that the disease didn't always cause the same symptoms, and some people never developed symptoms or didn't do so until later in life.

This combination of readily available antibody tests and increased awareness of the varying nature of the disease's symptoms has led to greater numbers of people being diagnosed with celiac disease.

Simply having the right genetic makeup, however, doesn't guarantee you'll develop celiac disease, just that the possibility is there. In places where celiac disease is more prevalent, estimates are that about a third of the population carries one of these specific genes. But only a small percentage of the carriers — about 2 to 5 percent — actually develop the disease. This is likely because HLA-DQ2 and HLA-DQ8 aren't the only key players involved. Other genes, in addition HLA-DQ2 and HLA-DQ8, are needed for the disease to occur. A number of studies looking at people with celiac disease and their relatives have identified other genes as potential contributors to the disease.

GLUTEN The other key ingredient necessary for celiac disease is exposure to gluten. If you never consumed gluten, you'd never develop celiac disease, even if you had a genetic susceptibility. But we know that's almost impossible. In many countries, including the United States, gluten-containing foods are everywhere. In fact, wheat-based cereals are a first food for almost every child who lives anywhere that wheat is abundant.

As a result, it's not surprising that celiac disease is more prevalent in places where wheat consumption is high, such as Europe, the Americas and Australia. But celiac disease has also been found in other locations such as Northern India, where people eat more wheat products than in Southern India, and in North Africa and the Middle East, where bulgur and couscous, both forms of wheat, are staple food items.

As food trends change around the world, celiac disease could become even more common globally. In many developing countries, Western-style diets that feature a much higher proportion of wheat-based products are becoming more popular. Experts expect that the number of people with celiac disease in these countries will increase with the change in diet.

TRIGGERING EVENT For some people, more than just the right genes and consuming gluten are needed for celiac disease to develop. Many people carry the specific HLA genes and they eat gluten, but they don't develop celiac disease. This has led researchers to conclude that in many circumstances another element is required, what's often called a triggering event. Sometimes, for reasons that aren't clear, celiac disease emerges after some form of trauma, such as an infection, physical injury, the stress of pregnancy, severe stress or surgery. How or why these conditions trigger the onset of celiac disease is unclear.

This may also be the reason why some people don't develop the disease until later in life. It's not uncommon for a person with celiac disease to look back and remember that it was after a specific event that he or she began to experience symptoms associated with the disease.

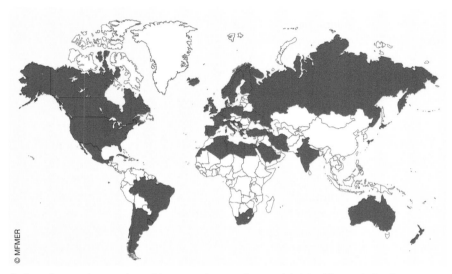

Celiac disease is now found in several countries worldwide. The red shading indicates countries where the disease is known to exist. Prevalence of the disease in these countries varies from approximately 0.5 percent of the population to more than 2 percent of the population.

Increasing numbers

Recent studies estimate the number of people worldwide with celiac disease is probably close to 1 percent of the general population. However, this number can vary substantially from country to country and among ethnic groups. In Europe, Finland has a higher than average prevalence of the disease, somewhere around 2 percent, whereas in Germany less than 0.5 percent of the population has celiac disease. In the United States, about 1 percent of the white population has celiac disease. In Mexico it's closer to 2 percent of the population.

It's also not uncommon for numbers to vary within regions. Denmark, for instance, has a remarkably lower prevalence than neighboring Sweden. In places such as China and Japan, it's rare for people to carry the genes associated with celiac disease, but in northwest Africa and the Middle East, prevalence is comparable to that of Western Europe and North America.

The number of people actually diagnosed with celiac disease, however, is less than 1 percent of the population. This is because people's symptoms may be minor or they don't fill the bill. In some cases, people have been told they have another condition when celiac disease is really at the root of the problem.

Studies conducted in defined populations of Americans as well as a rigorous sampling of people older than age 6 suggest that 1 in 141 Americans — approximately 1.8 million people — likely have celiac disease. Many have no symptoms or known risk factors and remain undiagnosed.

In other words, a lot of people may be walking around with celiac disease and not know it.

Are you at risk?

Celiac disease tends to occur more often in some groups than in others, although the degree of risk isn't the same for every group. For example, celiac disease is more often diagnosed in women than in men, but this is the case with a number of autoimmune disorders. And just because you're female doesn't mean you should be screened for celiac. On the other hand, relatives of people with celiac disease have a particularly high risk of having it, too.

Here are some of the factors that might put you at an increased risk of celiac disease.

FAMILY HISTORY If you have a relative with celiac disease, the chances are increased that you have the disease, too. This is because of the disease's genetic links. Several studies show that first-degree relatives of people with celiac disease are at a substantially increased risk of the disease.

The highest risk is among siblings. If you have celiac disease, your brothers or sisters have up to a 20 percent chance of having the disease as well. The risk is less for your parents or children. The risk is also less for second-degree relatives, such as your nieces or nephews, and your grandchildren.

Dermatitis herpetiformis, an itchy skin rash related to celiac disease, also runs in families. If one of your close relatives has this type of rash, you're at higher risk of developing dermatitis herpetiformis or celiac disease.

OTHER AUTOIMMUNE DISORDERS Celiac disease is associated with other autoimmune disorders, conditions in which the body attacks itself. They include:

- **Type 1 diabetes.** Type 1 diabetes results when your immune system mistakenly destroys insulin-producing cells in your pancreas, so your body doesn't produce enough insulin. Between 4 and 11 percent of people with type 1 diabetes have celiac disease.

- **Autoimmune thyroid disease.** This includes Hashimoto's disease and Graves' disease, conditions that affect the thyroid gland, leading to an underactive or overactive thyroid. People with these disorders are more likely to have celiac disease.

- ❋ **Sjögren's syndrome.** Sjögren's syndrome causes dry mouth and eyes. Reports indicate about 12 to 14 percent of people with Sjögren's syndrome also have celiac disease.

- ❋ **Microscopic colitis.** Also known as lymphocytic or collagenous colitis, this condition results from an inflammation of the large intestine (colon) that causes watery diarrhea. Your chances of developing celiac disease are greatly increased if you have microscopic colitis. People who have both conditions generally have more severe damage to intestinal villi and persistent diarrhea.

Genetic studies show that celiac disease and many of these disorders share certain HLA genes, suggesting similarities in their genetic profiles. However, more research is needed to clarify the relationship.

CHROMOSOME DISORDERS Having Down syndrome or Turner syndrome increases your risk of celiac disease. A recent report from Sweden indicated a sixfold increase in the risk of celiac disease among people with Down syndrome. However, it's still not exactly clear how the two are connected.

Turner syndrome is a condition affecting girls and women that results from a missing or incomplete sex chromosome. The condition is associated with various autoimmune disorders, including celiac disease. Estimates are that between 5 and 8 percent of girls and women with Turner syndrome also have celiac disease.

RACE AND ETHNICITY For a long time, celiac disease was only thought to occur in whites. But it can occur in people of other ethnic backgrounds, including those of Hispanic and Arab descents. In the United States, celiac disease is found predominantly in whites. It's reported to be less common in blacks, Hispanic-Americans and other minority groups.

However, a study conducted in Mexico found that celiac disease is quite common in that country, its prevalence similar to that of the United States. Other studies suggest that celiac disease may be underdiagnosed in some minority populations. It's not clear why these variations occur. It may have to do with genetics, dietary differences, geographical location, or awareness and testing practices.

What's changed?

Part of the reason celiac disease and gluten have become hot topics in recent years is because of the increase in people being diagnosed. Greater numbers of people who previously would have slipped under the radar are being told they have celiac disease. But improved diagnosis doesn't account for all of it. More people than ever before are developing the illness, and doctors are trying to determine why.

Increased rates in the United States in particular are illustrated in a study published by a group of doctors, some from Mayo Clinic, who analyzed a large collection of frozen blood samples drawn between 1948 and 1954. The samples were taken from healthy young Air Force recruits and had remained frozen in a research lab until they were moved to the University of Minnesota.

Researchers wanting to examine the prevalence of celiac disease over time tested the well-preserved blood samples for celiac disease. And then they compared the results with blood samples drawn from two present-day groups of volunteers: one, a group of older adults similar in age to what the recruits would currently have been, and two, a group of young adults similar in age to the Air Force men when they were tested.

What the researchers found was unexpected. Of the recruit blood samples, 1 in 652 were positive for celiac disease. Of the present-day older group, 1 in 121 had undiagnosed celiac disease, and in the present-day younger group, 1 out of every 106 persons had undiagnosed celiac disease. The prevalence of celiac disease had increased at least four times over the course of 50 to 60 years. Other studies conducted in the United States and in Europe also show that celiac disease is on the rise.

LOOKING FOR CLUES Since human genes evolve incredibly slowly, it seems likely that the answer isn't solely genetic. Chances are, other factors are behind the rate increase. Scientists are trying to tease out clues from ongoing research regarding what might be making celiac disease more prevalent than ever before. Here are a few of the theories being studied.

Introduction of gluten When and how gluten is introduced in early infancy may play a role. Studies suggest that breast-feeding while introducing infant cereal containing gluten into a baby's diet seems to have a protective effect. On the other hand, introducing gluten too early or too late — before 3 months of age or after 7 months — may increase a child's risk of celiac disease. Eating too much gluten early in life also may increase the risk.

Evidence to support these ideas comes from an "epidemic" of celiac disease that occurred in Sweden during the mid- to late 1980s and the early 1990s. Between 1985 and 1987, the number of infants diagnosed with celiac disease rose sharply then plateaued for a few years, followed by an abrupt drop in 1995 to previous levels.

What happened to cause this epidemic-like increase in celiac disease rates in these children? Researchers believe the answer may be related to the number of infants being fed formula that contained gluten, combined with a change in recommendations to delay the introduction of cereal and efforts to promote breast-feeding. The researchers concluded that no single trend seemed responsible for the steep rise and decline of celiac incidence rates, but a combination of factors may have made it easier for celiac disease to develop in these infants.

More sanitary environment Another theory, commonly called the "hygiene hypothesis," proposes that because our current environment is so much cleaner and more sanitary than in the past, the balance between microbes and the human immune system has been thrown off, making people with less exposure to infectious organisms more susceptible to autoimmune diseases, such as celiac disease.

In addition, researchers have found that celiac disease may be slightly more common in children delivered by cesarean section, suggesting that perhaps there's some protective effect from the exposure a child gets in the birth canal.

However, this is likely only a partial explanation because there's evidence that indicates early childhood infections, especially gastrointestinal ones, may actually increase the risk of celiac disease in children who are genetically predisposed to the condition. In addition, celiac disease is a health problem in some developing countries with poor sanitation, which counteracts the "hygiene hypothesis."

Changes in wheat and its uses Other theories revolve around changes instituted in the past few decades as to how wheat is grown, processed and consumed, and whether these changes may put genetically predisposed individuals at a greater risk of developing celiac disease. Because of ongoing cross-breeding of wheat cultures, we now have many different strains of wheat than those that existed even a few decades back. Have we changed wheat to make it less compatible to the human body and more difficult to digest?

Still much to learn

In the last few decades, we've amassed a great deal of knowledge about celiac disease and gluten, but there's still a great deal more to learn. Scientists continue to explore what factors — from genetics to environment to individual body systems — might contribute to the development of celiac disease. They also want to know more about why the manner in which the disease presents itself is changing. Why is it that what used to be a disease found primarily in malnourished children is now more often diagnosed in adults who appear to be well-nourished?

And then there's the issue of the millions of people who may have celiac disease and are unaware of it. A lot of discussion in health care circles these days revolves around the costs and benefits of screening people who don't have symptoms but who may be at risk of celiac disease and might benefit from treatment.

The next chapter takes a look at the many signs and symptoms of celiac disease. You'll better understand why people often live with the disease for years before finally receiving a diagnosis.

CHAPTER TWO

Signs that something's wrong

Millions of people may be walking around with celiac disease right now and not realize it. Part of the reason is that the disease acts in strange ways. Most people equate celiac disease with abdominal cramps, diarrhea and weight loss. That makes sense because the disease begins in and damages the small intestine. But what you may not know — and what surprises many people — is that celiac disease can affect almost every part of your body, triggering literally hundreds of symptoms.

Unlike other illnesses in which the disease's progression follows a similar script from one person to the next, the storylines of people with celiac disease are often different. One person might feel bloated and gassy, another might experience headaches and fatigue. Some people have difficulty trying to keep weight on, while others are overweight. And to thicken the plot: Quite a few people don't experience any symptoms at all.

As you read through this chapter, you may recognize symptoms you've been experiencing that you didn't realize could be celiac disease. Don't feel guilty or feel that you've messed up somehow. You haven't. Because of the varied way it expresses itself, the disease is easy to miss.

In this chapter, we organize the signs and symptoms of celiac disease according to how and where they affect your body. Doctors, however, have other ways of classifying celiac symptoms that help them sort through the ins and outs of the disorder. You may hear your doctor use the following terms when talking about celiac disease:

Classical celiac disease. This is the name used when the main symptoms are indications of malabsorption — chronic or intermittent diarrhea; pale, fatty stools; weight loss; and failure to thrive in children. These symptoms were once considered "typical," but because the way celiac disease presents itself has changed in recent years, they aren't really the most common signs and symptoms anymore. So classical is the preferred name.

Nonclassical celiac disease. Also known as atypical celiac disease, nonclassical disease doesn't include signs and symptoms of malabsorption. Instead, the individual may have abdominal pain, constipation, fatigue or anemia.

Asymptomatic celiac disease. Another name for this type is silent celiac disease. It refers to people who don't seem to be experiencing any symptoms. Individuals with asymptomatic disease are often diagnosed through screening programs for people at high risk, generally because they have close relatives with celiac disease.

Potential celiac disease. Sometimes referred to as latent celiac disease, this type is used to describe people without symptoms who are considered at high risk of developing the disease later in life. The lining of the small intestine looks normal but blood tests are positive for celiac disease.

Subclinical celiac disease. This term is sometimes used to describe mild or seemingly unrelated signs and symptoms that aren't normally associated with celiac disease, but may be tied to the condition because of other factors that raise suspicion an individual may have celiac disease.

Terms doctors use to describe different types of celiac disease

Signs and symptoms of celiac disease

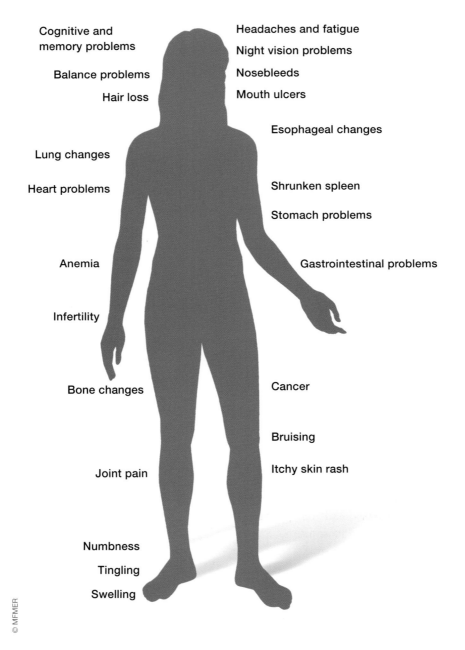

Cognitive and memory problems

Balance problems

Hair loss

Lung changes

Heart problems

Anemia

Infertility

Bone changes

Joint pain

Numbness

Tingling

Swelling

Headaches and fatigue

Night vision problems

Nosebleeds

Mouth ulcers

Esophageal changes

Shrunken spleen

Stomach problems

Gastrointestinal problems

Cancer

Bruising

Itchy skin rash

© MFMER

Almost all parts of the body may be affected by celiac disease. The disease presents itself in many different ways. This is why celiac disease is often difficult to recognize.

Even doctors don't always recognize the signs and symptoms, and it's easy to attribute many of the characteristics of celiac disease to other conditions, such as irritable bowel syndrome or skin allergies.

And if you're thinking, "My symptoms aren't that bad. I'm not going to worry about it," think again. The truth is, untreated celiac disease can lead to serious health concerns, which is why diagnosis and treatment are so important. In addition to conditions such as anemia and osteoporosis, untreated celiac disease is associated with cancers of the digestive tract and lymph glands. The bottom line is this: If you think you could have celiac disease or your biological relatives have been diagnosed with the illness, see your doctor and get checked out. Don't wait until the disease causes significant damage.

This chapter looks at some of the more common signs and symptoms of celiac disease. But keep in mind that the illness can express itself in many different ways and is associated with many different conditions. Talk to your doctor if you have further questions or you're wondering if what you're experiencing might be related to celiac disease.

Digestive problems

People sometimes find it difficult to talk about symptoms associated with digestive problems. This may include symptoms such as diarrhea, gas or abdominal cramps. Though not everyone with celiac disease experiences these problems, they're often the most well-recognized indications of the disease.

When the small intestine is damaged, it can't properly absorb nutrients such as fat, carbohydrates, protein and electrolytes. This can wreak havoc on normal gastrointestinal functions and lead to various symptoms.

DIARRHEA AND ABNORMAL STOOLS It's not uncommon for people with celiac disease to have regular bouts of diarrhea, mushy stools or bulky stools that float due to large amounts of unabsorbed fat. In addition, the bowel movements can be very odorous. People with celiac disease will often say that family members made fun of them for "stinking up the place."

The diarrhea and abnormal stools result from malabsorption. Unabsorbed nutrients add to the stool's bulk and pull in liquid from the intestinal lining, making the stool more watery and bulky. The bad odor that accompanies the bowel movements comes from not being able to absorb fat. The fat stays in the intestine and becomes part of your stool, a condition known as steatorrhea.

Unabsorbed fat also makes you want to empty your bowels more often. For some people, diarrhea is a real problem and they feel like they spend the entire day on the toilet. Some report having 10 or more bowel movements a day. Others find they're not bothered as severely or as often.

Interestingly, a few people with celiac disease experience the complete opposite. Instead of diarrhea, they're bothered by constipation. Malabsorption of nutrients, inflammation in the gut, and nervous system and hormone changes may cause your bowels to operate more sluggishly than normal.

PAIN AND BLOATING Many people with celiac disease experience belly pain, bloating and excessive gas (flatulence). Digestion may be noisy, causing lots of rumbling sounds due to excess gas and liquid in your intestine. Sugars and fats that don't get absorbed can draw fluid into your intestine from your body causing the small intestine to swell up. When unabsorbed nutrients such as carbohydrates arrive in your colon, bacteria that reside in your colon break down (ferment) these nutrients. The fermentation process creates large amounts of gas, which can make you feel bloated and uncomfortable, and results in excessive flatulence.

Damage to your small intestine also can make it more difficult for you to digest milk and other dairy products. That's why a number of people with celiac disease are also lactose intolerant. Lactose intolerance, in turn, can contribute to diarrhea, pain and bloating.

HEARTBURN Some people with celiac disease are bothered by heartburn, or gastroesophageal reflux disease (GERD). One study found that, before treatment,

A double whammy: Troubles with gluten and lactose

If you have celiac disease, you may be surprised to find out you're also lactose intolerant. Isn't the true culprit behind your discomfort gluten? Yes, gluten is the bad guy, but the damage it does to your small intestine can make it difficult for you to digest other foods, such as dairy products.

Cells located at the tips of the hairlike projections that line your small intestine (villi) produce the enzyme lactase. This enzyme helps you digest milk sugar (lactose) in the foods you eat, mainly dairy products. When the villi are damaged from celiac disease, the cells aren't able to produce lactase as they normally would, making you lactose intolerant as well.

Once you remove gluten from your diet so your small intestine can heal, villi generally grow back and the production of lactase often returns to normal. With time, you may find yourself able to drink milk and eat some dairy foods again.

30 percent of people with celiac disease reported moderate to severe symptoms of heartburn, compared with only 6 percent of people without celiac disease.

The exact mechanism by which the condition can lead to heartburn isn't clear, but it usually goes away after starting a gluten-free diet. It may be how food moves out of the stomach, causing a backup of acid.

Skin and hair problems

Sometimes celiac disease reveals itself by way of hair loss or a skin disorder. Hair loss may be due to a zinc deficiency or to a change in the normal pattern of hair loss so that all hair is lost at once instead of gradually over a period of time. More commonly, celiac disease is linked to skin rash. Sometimes celiac disease makes itself known by way of a skin condition known as dermatitis herpetiformis.

DERMATITIS HERPETIFORMIS Dermatitis herpetiformis is an intensely itchy, blistering skin rash that's found mainly on your elbows, forearms, back, knees, scalp or buttocks (see page 38). The rash may come and go, but rarely does it resolve for good. Dermatitis herpetiformis is fairly common. It occurs in about 1 out of every 10 or 20 people with celiac disease. The rash most commonly first develops around ages 40 to 50, but it can occur at any age.

People who have dermatitis herpetiformis typically don't have any gastro-intestinal symptoms, although they eventually experience changes to the lining of the small intestine identical to those of celiac disease. Dermatitis herpetiformis also carries other similar risks, such as development of other autoimmune diseases.

To treat the rash, the oral antibiotic dapsone is often prescribed. A topical steroid may improve the rash, but it won't do anything for intestinal damage. A gluten-free diet is necessary to remove the root cause of the rash and keep it from coming back, as well as to prevent future complications of celiac disease.

Oral and dental issues

Another place that celiac disease can show up is in your mouth. People with celiac disease tend to get canker sores inside their mouths more often than do people who don't have the disease. Canker sores can be a painful nuisance, but once you treat the disease, you likely won't get them as often.

A smooth tongue (atrophic glossitis) caused by deterioration of the small bumps on your tongue may leave your tongue inflamed and painful. This could be related to low levels of iron, folic acid or vitamin B-12. Painful cracking of the corners of the mouth may result from an iron deficiency.

Dermatitis herpetiformis

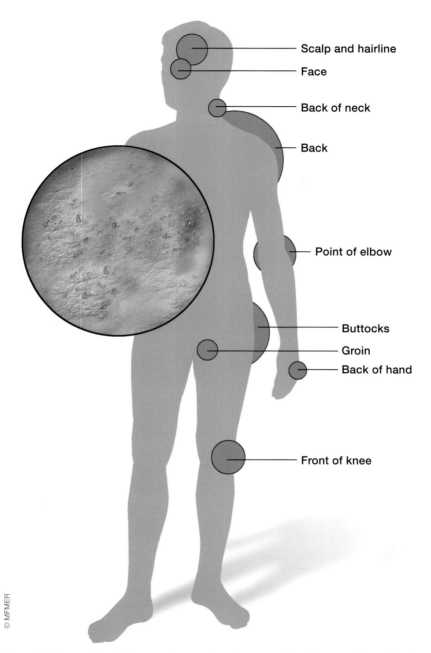

- Scalp and hairline
- Face
- Back of neck
- Back
- Point of elbow
- Buttocks
- Groin
- Back of hand
- Front of knee

© MFMER

Dermatitis herpetiformis is sometimes referred to as celiac disease of the skin. A gluten-free diet will clear the rash; however, healing often occurs slowly.

Celiac disease can also affect normal development of tooth enamel. This may be because not enough calcium is being absorbed during a child's early years to produce strong teeth. The damage may also be a direct result of the disease itself. Dental problems may not come to light until young adulthood. Some people go through a lot of restorative dental care before finally being diagnosed with celiac disease.

Brain and nervous system disorders

Researchers are finding that in a growing number of people, celiac disease doesn't cause gastrointestinal symptoms, but instead it manifests itself through brain and nervous system disorders.

Vitamin and mineral deficiencies related to malabsorption can certainly have a detrimental effect on the brain and nervous system. But some experts believe that the neurological symptoms connected to celiac disease may also be caused by an inappropriate immune response to gluten that damages brain and nerve cells, similar to what happens in the small intestine. Or it could be that these symptoms tend to occur in conjunction with celiac disease, but they aren't caused by it.

HEADACHES It's not unusual for people who've just been diagnosed with celiac disease to describe having migraine-like headaches. The headaches may be mild and happen every now and then, or they can be severely debilitating and frequent.

Studies examining brain images of people with celiac disease and a history of headaches show an association between the headaches and bright white spots on the brain, indicating damaged or abnormal areas. Once celiac disease is treated, the headaches typically go away. The white spots don't disappear, but treatment of celiac disease seems to stop them from developing.

NUMBNESS AND TINGLING Numbness and tingling in your feet and legs and later on your hands (peripheral neuropathy) are a common nerve-related symptom of celiac disease. The symptoms usually come on gradually, and they tend to happen every now and again and can't be easily explained by another condition. The numbness and tingling will generally disappear on a gluten-free diet, but the response may be very slow, taking months to years to completely correct.

Because many conditions can cause similar nervous system symptoms, it's not an easy jump from having numbness and tingling in your legs to suspecting you have celiac disease. The average amount of time between the onset of neuropathy and a diagnosis of celiac disease is about nine years.

GLUTEN ATAXIA Celiac disease is also associated with other neurological problems. Deficiencies in certain vitamins that can occur with celiac disease — in particular vitamin B-12, vitamin B-6, vitamin E and copper — may affect various nervous system functions. In addition to numbness and tingling in the feet and hands, the deficiencies can produce signs and symptoms such as a decline in hand coordination, difficulties with balance and walking, as well as generalized loss of strength. The word *ataxia* means without coordination. Some vitamin deficiencies can affect cognitive function and contribute to fatigue.

In addition to nutrient deficiencies, immune-related disorders generated by gluten may be misdirected against parts of the nervous system, producing neurological difficulties.

It's not clear exactly how celiac disease leads to ataxia. MRI scans reveal shrinkage of the brain's cerebellum in more than half the people with gluten

You don't have to be skinny to have celiac disease

Many people who are at a normal weight or who are overweight don't think they can have celiac disease because they weigh too much. This belief is even held by some doctors. People typically associate celiac disease with someone who's skinny and perhaps malnourished. For many years, this was the picture of celiac disease. But as the disease evolved — along with our awareness of its varied symptoms — it became clear that celiac disease doesn't occur only in people who are underweight.

In general, people with celiac disease may be thinner than the general population, but a substantial proportion are obese. In fact, a greater percentage of people with celiac disease are overweight than underweight. One analysis of close to 400 people with celiac disease found that while just over half of them were at a normal weight, only 5 percent were underweight and close to 40 percent were overweight. Similar results have been found in other studies.

How does this happen if essential nutrients including fat are supposedly sliding right through your intestine and into the toilet? The answer probably has to do with the patchy nature of celiac disease. Celiac disease primarily affects the upper portions of the small intestine known as the ataxia. The cerebellum is located in the lower part of the brain and controls involuntary muscle movement. It may be that your immune system, triggered by gluten ingestion, mistakenly attacks your cerebellum, destroying cells.

Prompt treatment can improve or stabilize symptoms. However, the longer the disease continues untreated, the harder it becomes to reverse the damage. A person with ataxia may not recover completely.

SEIZURES Seizures and epilepsy are associated with celiac disease, but the link is controversial. In fact, recent studies of large groups of people have noted that the incidence of epilepsy among people with celiac disease is actually about the same as the general population. In rare instances, celiac disease has been linked to excess calcium in the brain associated with seizures. The presence of celiac disease in a patient with seizures is important because it might affect absorption of certain medications.

duodenum and jejunum (see page 23). Damage to the tiny villi in the jejunum make absorption difficult in this portion of the intestine. Your lower small intestine (ileum), meanwhile, may not be as damaged and it adapts by taking on the role of its upper neighbor. Villi in the ileum, which normally digest and absorb mostly liquids, expand and grow bigger to absorb the extra nutrients coming through that weren't absorbed upstream.

So, even though you have celiac disease, you may still be eating and absorbing enough nutrients to prevent signs and symptoms of malabsorption, including weight loss.

In addition, sometimes the body senses it's short on certain micronutrients that aren't getting absorbed in the upper intestine because of damage to the villi. This feeling of being undernourished can drive a person to eat more food in an attempt to get more of the missing nutrients. But what can happen is that the nutrients still go unabsorbed but the extra calories are absorbed, causing weight gain.

Once gluten is eliminated from your diet and the upper intestine has a chance to heal, the lower intestine typically returns to normal. As a result, you're absorbing more nutrients than ever before, which is important to your health. However, this can lead to increased weight gain if you eat a lot of foods rich in calories. This is another reason why it's important to get help from a dietitian when starting on a gluten-free diet. You don't want your change in diet to cause an unwelcomed increase in weight.

Fatigue and mood disorders

Sometimes, symptoms associated with celiac disease can be more vague or subtle in nature. You may feel like you're in a fog or just plain "out of it." These symptoms might include feelings of tiredness, depression, irritability or anxiety. And they can sometimes seem more bothersome than other symptoms.

FATIGUE Fatigue is a common complaint of people diagnosed with celiac disease. People will often describe a feeling of being tired all of the time, despite getting enough sleep. Some people can't muster the energy to get through the day, and they aren't able to perform more-complex tasks.

Many factors can cause fatigue. It's possible that low levels of vitamins and other nutrients may contribute to fatigue, particularly B-12, B-6 and folic acid. In addition, a majority of adults with celiac disease have low iron levels (iron deficiency anemia). A celiac-damaged gut may not be able to absorb enough iron. Without adequate iron, your body can't produce enough hemoglobin, a substance in red blood cells that enables the cells to transport oxygen throughout your body. As a result, iron deficiency anemia can leave you feeling tired and short of breath. This may contribute to the fatigue commonly experienced by people with celiac disease. A thyroid disorder associated with celiac disease also may lead to fatigue.

Other causes of fatigue include depression, anxiety and lack of sleep. These conditions can result from worry about not knowing what's wrong with your body, or from the stress of learning how to manage celiac disease after it's been diagnosed. Muscle-related fatigue or severe fatigue may be related to other disorders that can accompany celiac disease, such as an endocrine or adrenal disorder.

DEPRESSION AND ANXIETY A substantial number of people with celiac disease say they feel depressed or anxious. But it's more difficult to determine whether these symptoms are connected to the disease process itself or whether they're due to the stress of coping with a lifelong illness.

For example, depression doesn't always improve after changing your diet. In fact, at first, adjusting to a completely new lifestyle can even add to feelings of being out of sorts or anxious. After a while, though, many people do begin to feel better and more in control of their lives.

Brain changes related to celiac disease may affect mood and behaviors. In addition to evidence indicating shrinking of the brain's cerebellum among some people with celiac disease, MRI scans also showed loss of grey matter in brain areas related to decision-making and psychomotor skills, similar to what's been found in people with depression. This suggests that depression may be at least partly related to the celiac disease process itself.

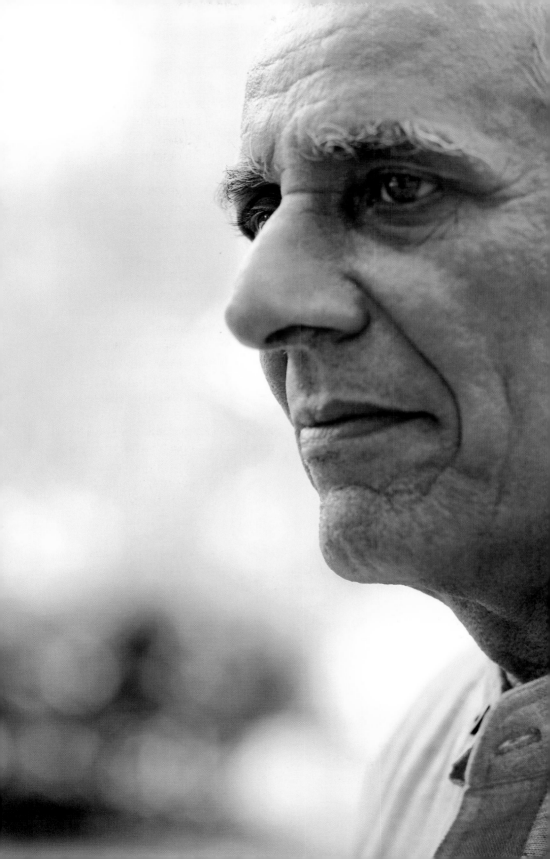

Whether emotional symptoms are a function of celiac disease or they result from having a chronic illness, it's not all in your head. The symptoms are real and deserve attention. Sometimes, they can become a barrier to treatment.

Bone and joint problems

When your small intestine is damaged, your body may not be able to absorb calcium and other bone-building nutrients. One way celiac disease is sometimes diagnosed is with the emergence of bone and joint problems.

BONES People with celiac disease may have thinning and weakening of their bones due to low bone mineral density. Studies suggest that among adults with celiac disease, about a third have bone mineral density that's less than ideal (osteopenia), and another third have serious bone loss (osteoporosis).

Your bones are in a constant state of renewal — new bone is made and old bone is broken down. When you're young, your body makes new bone faster than it breaks down old bone and your bone mass increases. Most people reach their peak bone mass by their late 20s. As you age, you lose bone mass faster than you create it. Calcium and vitamin D are important to this process of bone remodeling.

With celiac disease, the damage that occurs in your small intestine can prevent you from absorbing calcium and vitamin D needed to maintain strong bones. Immune system and inflammatory changes associated with celiac disease also may contribute to bone loss. And because many people with celiac disease are lactose intolerant (see page 36), they aren't consuming as many dairy products. This also can contribute to calcium and vitamin D deficiencies.

Not only is bone density reduced, an increase in fractures often occurs in individuals with celiac disease. This increased fracture risk may persist after the diagnosis and treatment of celiac disease, especially among adults who aren't able to fully recover a loss of bone mass. This can also be an issue for people who've had celiac disease since they were children and didn't achieve the peak bone mass they should have.

A gluten-free diet will often improve celiac-related bone loss. Adults, however, generally don't recover as much bone mass as do children treated at a young age, when they still have time to build bone. While on a gluten-free diet, make sure you're getting enough calcium and vitamin D. Exercise is important, and in some cases osteoporosis medications may be appropriate.

JOINTS Aching, painful joints can be another symptom of celiac disease. Typically, pain occurs in the hands, shoulders, elbows, wrists or knees, and sometimes in the spine and hips. The pain may come and go for a few weeks at a time, and it may resemble the pain of arthritis. Experts have even wondered whether people with arthritis should be screened for celiac disease.

Studies looking at the connection between celiac disease and joint pain and arthritis are limited, but they generally support the idea that there is a link. One study, for example, found arthritis in just over 25 percent of people with celiac disease. As further proof, joint pain and swelling among people with celiac disease don't always respond to corticosteroids, a conventional arthritis treatment, but do seem to improve in response to a gluten-free diet.

It's possible that the inflammation associated with celiac disease might affect your joints, making them inflamed and achy. Also, since one autoimmune disease tends to increase your risk of another, it's also possible the joint pain may be caused by rheumatoid arthritis, an autoimmune-related form of arthritis that produces inflammation in the joints.

Hormone issues

Celiac disease can affect hormone production in your body and disrupt reproductive functions. As with many other symptoms of celiac disease, it's uncertain whether these kinds of reproductive changes are caused by possible nutritional deficiencies associated with celiac disease or whether they're an effect of an immune system that's out of whack.

ABNORMAL MENSTRUATION AND INFERTILITY In women, celiac disease can lead to abnormal menstrual patterns. Among teenage girls, possible signs of celiac disease include menstruation beginning later than normal or having irregular periods or loss of periods.

Celiac disease has also been diagnosed in women with unexplained infertility and in women who've had frequent miscarriages. A couple having difficulty getting pregnant may each be tested for celiac disease as part of his or her medical evaluation.

Treating celiac disease can help regulate hormones and menstrual patterns, improving a woman's chances of getting pregnant. This can help avoid more involved and often expensive fertility treatments. In addition, untreated celiac disease can have a harmful effect on pregnancy. Malabsorption of vitamins and minerals can increase a pregnant woman's chance of having complications, such as the baby being born too early or with a low birth weight.

MALE CONCERNS Celiac disease can also affect male fertility. Evidence suggests that among men with celiac disease, the shape and quality of their sperm may be altered, or they may have fewer sperm than normal. These problems generally correct themselves once celiac disease is treated.

Celiac disease may also affect regulation of the hypothalamus and pituitary glands, organs involved in the production of hormones, causing testosterone and other male hormones to reach abnormal levels.

Other conditions

Celiac disease is also associated with a number of other disorders. Additional ways the disease may present itself include vision problems, such as night vision difficulties, dry eyes or inflammation. The disease can also produce unexplained nosebleeds, bruising and swelling (edema).

Additional conditions linked to the disease include lung disorders such as fibrosis and sarcoidosis and stomach problems such as atrophic gastritis. The disease may also produce a shrunken spleen.

In rare instances, celiac disease may trigger heart-related conditions, such as cardiomyopathy, myocarditis or an autoimmune reaction to the muscle of the heart, similar to that of the small intestine.

Test abnormalities

In some cases, celiac disease doesn't produce any obvious signs or symptoms except for abnormalities that show up in routine blood tests.

A blood test may show iron deficiency anemia. For example, you go to donate blood but are refused because your iron level is low. Many conditions can cause anemia, however, and a doctor may not associate it with celiac disease. This may be especially true in women whose low iron levels may be blamed on blood loss from heavy periods. A clue that iron deficiency anemia may be linked to celiac disease is when it's hard to treat, even with supplements, because of malabsorption in the small intestine.

People with celiac disease may also experience abnormal results on liver function tests. Blood tests may show mildly elevated levels of aspartate aminotransferase (AST) and alanine aminotransferase (ALT) in the liver. Increases of these enzymes that can't be explained by another condition may be related to celiac disease.

Dangers of the disease

If your symptoms are mild or you aren't experiencing symptoms, you may wonder why you need to be tested or make significant changes to your diet. For some people, it can be easy to brush off the disease. But celiac disease is a condition that can't be ignored. If left undiagnosed and untreated, it can lead to serious complications, some which can be life-threatening.

Kids and celiac disease

Celiac disease in children may present itself a little differently than it does in adults. Adults generally have signs and symptoms that are mild and nongastrointestinal in nature, such as anemia, fatigue or headaches. Kids, especially very young children, are more likely to have classic signs and symptoms of celiac disease: belly pain, chronic or intermittent diarrhea, a swollen (distended) belly, and failure to grow or gain weight at the same rate as their peers. A child's growth curve may fall off the usual growth pattern.

It's not uncommon, however, for children to experience symptoms that are nongastrointestinal, especially as they get older. Feeling irritable or lethargic is common in children with celiac disease, and adolescents may experience depression or panic attacks.

It's also not unusual for celiac disease to show up in kids' teeth. Enamel on their permanent teeth — especially the incisors and first molars — may be underdeveloped, allowing the teeth to erode. This can create patches of yellowish-brown discoloration and shallow grooves or pits. In some cases, the shape of the tooth may even change so that the tips become sharp and pointy. Problems such as these are generally an indication to get tested for celiac disease.

Another indication of celiac disease can be frequent broken bones. Because of the damage to their small intestines, children with celiac disease often don't absorb enough calcium and vitamin D, which can result in lower bone mineral density than normal for their ages. This can lead to soft, thin bones (osteomalacia) that break more easily.

The effect of celiac disease on hormone production also can result in short stature and delayed puberty in adolescents. The good news is children with celiac disease who start a gluten-free diet before they complete puberty may still reach their full height, even if they were shorter than normal beforehand.

Not all childhood disorders linked to celiac disease have been proven. Some researchers have suggested a possible association between celiac disease and behavioral disorders in children, such as learning disabilities, attention-deficit/hyperactivity disorder (ADHD) and autism. Increased diagnoses of autism and greater awareness of gluten sensitivity have indeed led many parents to wonder whether gluten might play a role in these disorders. While some observational reports have suggested that a gluten-free diet may improve behavior and cognitive skills in children with autism, there's not enough scientific data to support a strong connection. Further research is needed to clarify if there truly is a link between gluten and behavioral disorders in children.

CANCER People with celiac disease have a greater risk of developing intestinal lymphoma and other types of digestive cancers compared with the general population.

Risk of cancer appears to be increased if symptoms are more severe or if the disease has gone undiagnosed for a long period of time, resulting in nutritional deficiencies. However, other evidence suggests the risk may be tied to the inflammatory nature of celiac disease and not to gluten exposure, since a number of other inflammatory disorders also carry an increased risk of cancer. Interestingly, women with celiac disease have a reduced risk of breast cancer.

While information regarding cancer risk is not clear-cut, most experts support the idea that adhering to a gluten-free diet can reduce your risk of certain cancers. Regular monitoring for cancer may not be necessary, unless symptoms warrant it.

OTHER AUTOIMMUNE DISORDERS There is controversy as to whether celiac disease is merely associated with other autoimmune diseases or whether untreated celiac disease and continued gluten exposure increases the risk of other autoimmune diseases. Evidence shows that people with celiac disease develop other autoimmune disorders more frequently than do people who don't have celiac disease.

Some autoimmune disorders associated with celiac disease include type I diabetes, autoimmune thyroid disease, Sjögren's syndrome — a disorder that causes dry mouth and eyes — and microscopic colitis, an inflammatory disorder of the large intestine. As with the risk of cancer, it's still up in the air as to whether the association with other autoimmune disorders is linked to gluten or to the immune system. It's also possible that other autoimmune diseases occur with celiac disease because they share the same genetic and environmental triggers for the disease.

Most of the time, if celiac disease is diagnosed early and gluten is promptly removed from the diet, the majority of complications can be prevented and a person with celiac disease can live just as well and long as someone with no illness.

Now what?

As you can see, celiac disease can cause any number of signs and symptoms ranging from more-obvious gastrointestinal problems to more-subtle nuisances such as headaches, depression or anemia. It's also true that many of these symptoms are common to a host of other disorders.

So how do you know if you have celiac disease or not? The next chapter can help you assess your health to determine if your symptoms may be linked to celiac disease. If you think you may have celiac disease or you're simply not sure, the first step is to talk with your doctor about it. He or she can review your symptoms and run initial screening tests to determine if you might be at risk of the disease and should have further testing.

If it turns out you do have celiac disease, treatment with a gluten-free diet can help you feel much better and help prevent many of the problems associated with celiac disease.

CHAPTER THREE

Do you have celiac disease?

It may be that until recently you'd never heard of celiac disease. But now that you've read through the range of symptoms associated with the disease, some of them sound a little familiar. You've dealt with gastrointestinal discomfort for much of your life, but you always thought it was due to something else or that was just how things were for you. Or maybe you've always felt fatigued and low on energy, but you just assumed it was your busy lifestyle. And the regular headaches? Par for the course.

It can be easy to ignore these common signs and symptoms or chalk them up to everyday occurrences, but that's not a good idea. Although celiac disease can cause a host of different symptoms — some of which may sound an awful lot like those associated with irritable bowel syndrome, migraines or chronic fatigue — once it's suspected, it's a disease that can be fairly easily diagnosed. And it can effectively be treated.

If you're wondering if you could have celiac disease, this chapter can help you assess your situation and decide whether it might be time to bring up the disease and possible testing with your doctor. While it's true that not every discomfort is a sign of illness, frequent distress that doesn't respond to conventional treatments needs to be attended to.

Unfortunately, many people live with celiac disease for many years before it's diagnosed. They don't think their symptoms are that bad, they attribute them to something else, or their doctors don't test for the disease.

10 common myths

Many people don't think it's possible they could have celiac disease because they don't fill the bill — they're not underweight, they don't have diarrhea, and they're not Irish. Misinformation abounds when it comes to celiac disease, partly because outdated information is hard to root out. Part of determining if you might have celiac disease, is sorting out fact from fiction.

MYTH 1: I was born with celiac disease.
Although you might be born with a genetic susceptibility to celiac disease, the condition doesn't develop until you ingest gluten, and perhaps not even then. Some people develop celiac disease within the first year of life when they start eating gluten found in infant cereal. Others don't develop it until their adult years — the disease can develop even in late adulthood. And still others never seem to be affected by it, even though they carry the required genes and they eat gluten. It's not clear why some people develop celiac disease and most others don't, even though they're genetically predisposed. Why the timing of onset can differ so much from one person to the next is another million-dollar question.

MYTH 2: I'm too fat or too tall to have celiac disease.
Signs of malnutrition, such as being underweight or much shorter than your peers, are considered to be classic signs of celiac disease. This happens when vital nutrients pass through the digestive tract unabsorbed because of severe damage to the small intestine. But the disease and its diagnosis have evolved in such a way that malnutrition is no longer the primary sign of celiac disease. In fact, some people with celiac disease are actually overweight, even obese. Tall people can have the disease, too.

MYTH 3: Only Irish people get celiac disease.
This is another frequent misconception. Celiac disease was once considered most common in people of Irish ancestry. However, recent population studies have shown that celiac disease is found in places all over the world, with the possible exception of countries in East Asia and sub-Saharan Africa. Within the U.S., celiac disease may be more common among whites than among people of other races or ethnicities, but more research is required. There are gaps in knowledge that need to be filled to get a more complete picture of the disease's prevalence in the U.S. and globally.

MYTH 4: No one in my family has celiac disease, so I can't have it.
While celiac disease often runs in families, in at least half of cases only one family member has the disease. If your parents don't have celiac disease that

isn't a guarantee you don't have it. The disease can skip generations and the interplay of genetics and other risk factors is complex.

MYTH 5: It's not celiac disease because I don't have chronic diarrhea.
People often think they can't have celiac disease because they don't have any problems with diarrhea. The truth is, only around half of adults with celiac disease have chronic diarrhea. Others have other gastrointestinal symptoms such as feeling bloated after meals, heartburn or even constipation. In addition, it's not uncommon for people with celiac disease to have few, if any digestive problems, but instead they have anemia, fatigue, skin rashes, headaches, or numbness in their hands or feet.

MYTH 6: If it doesn't bother me, it's OK to eat it.
If you have celiac disease, it may take only a few microscopic gluten particles to set off an immune reaction that can inflame and damage your gut. Sensitivity to ingestion of gluten varies among individuals. However, inflammatory changes in the intestine don't always correlate directly with gastrointestinal symptoms. So even though you might feel fine, that doesn't mean that damage isn't occurring. The more damage that occurs and the longer the small intestine remains unhealed, the greater the complications that may develop, such as osteoporosis or intestinal cancer.

MYTH 7: If it makes me sick, it must have gluten in it.
When your intestine is damaged, even when you eat foods that don't contain gluten you can still experience symptoms. The inflammation in your small intestine makes it difficult to digest certain foods. One example is lactose in dairy products. Often times, people with celiac disease are lactose intolerant as well.

MYTH 8: If it's gluten-free, it's good for me.
Just because something is gluten-free doesn't automatically make it healthy, especially when it comes to processed foods. In fact, gluten-free products may be less healthy if they're low in fiber or made with nonfortified ingredients that don't contain the same amount of vitamins and minerals that wheat-containing products do. In addition, they may be high in fat or sugar in an effort to make up for any lack of flavor or texture.

   When following a gluten-free diet, you still need to make sure that it adheres to the basic rules of healthy eating. Whole foods such as fruits and vegetables that are naturally gluten-free and also abundant in antioxidants, vitamins and other essential nutrients are a great choice for anyone. And there are a variety of healthy whole grains that don't contain gluten, such as rice, corn, quinoa and buckwheat, to name a few. But when it comes to processed foods, it's still important to read the nutrition label, regardless of whether it says it's gluten-free or not.

MYTH 9: I can't touch anything with gluten in it.
An immune reaction occurs only when you eat gluten and the gluten interacts with your immune system. Making a sandwich for your child or cooking pasta won't cause a problem unless you eat the food. However, cross-contamination of gluten-free foods can occur if you use the same knife to cut your apple as you did to slice your son's sandwich.

By the same token, gluten-containing skin care products and cosmetics generally aren't a problem unless you accidentally swallow a large amount. To be safe, you may want to avoid using products that contain gluten on your lips or around your mouth, such as certain types of lip balm, lipstick, mouthwash and toothpaste. If you're uncertain whether a product contains gluten, you may need to contact the manufacturer.

Some people develop a form of celiac disease called dermatitis herpetiformis, which causes an itchy, blistering rash. This skin disorder is also linked to gluten and is also caused by ingesting gluten, not by skin contact with gluten.

MYTH 10: I can outgrow celiac disease.
Celiac disease is a lifelong condition — a permanent, genetically based aversion to gluten. In some children, the disease may seem to go away or become "silent" during the teen years, but problems may surface again later in life, so it's important to continue treating it. If it's truly celiac disease, you can't outgrow it.

A difficult disease to identify

One factor that stands out when it comes to celiac disease is the length of time between when a person starts to feel symptoms and when he or she is finally diagnosed as having celiac disease. Some estimates are that it takes an average of 11 years before a person with symptoms is accurately diagnosed with the disease. So why does it take so long for people to learn they have celiac disease? There are a lot of reasons.

SIMILARITIES TO OTHER DISEASES It's not uncommon for people with celiac disease to be diagnosed with the wrong condition. Because the disease's symptoms are similar to many other disorders, a doctor may attribute the symptoms to another condition and not think to check for celiac disease. Or you might even diagnose yourself and never bother to bring it up with your doctor because you think you can handle it on your own or that it's not a big deal.

Celiac disease is often mistaken for irritable bowel syndrome (IBS). That's no surprise, really, since IBS produces signs and symptoms very much like those of celiac disease — abdominal pain, bloating, gas and diarrhea. In fact, the two conditions are quite different. Celiac disease affects your small intestine and can actually cause tissue damage. IBS can affect both your small and large intestine (colon). It disrupts the function of your bowel but doesn't cause any visible damage.

While there are specific tests to diagnose celiac disease, an IBS diagnosis is made by excluding other possible causes. If you and your doctor don't rule out celiac disease, it may be missed entirely and it may be years before you reach an answer to your health problems. Because the cause of IBS isn't known, treatment is aimed primarily at managing symptoms, such as relieving diarrhea or constipation with lifestyle changes, medications or both. With celiac disease, removing gluten from your diet will eliminate most gastrointestinal symptoms within a matter of weeks.

Other conditions also can mask an underlying gluten problem if celiac disease isn't ruled out. Examples include chronic fatigue syndrome, fibromyalgia or unexplained nerve inflammation (idiopathic neuropathy).

LACK OF AWARENESS Although celiac disease is a hot topic these days, it was only a few years ago that the disease was considered rare in the U.S. Today, most people still know very little about the disease and are unaware that a key ingredient in bread and pasta can cause a lifelong illness.

VARIED SYMPTOMS Celiac disease has a chameleon-like nature. The way it presents itself can change from one person to the next. The wide range of signs and symptoms — from bellyaches to headaches to feelings of tingling and numbness — can be very confusing, not just for you but for your doctor as well. Plus, the symptoms are sometimes mild enough that people don't feel a need to see a doctor. A daily headache or a little gas after eating seems normal.

DIFFICULT TOPIC Let's face it, a lot of people have difficulty talking about things like bowel movements and excessive gas. If your doctor doesn't ask about issues such as stomach cramps or bowel movements, you may be reluctant to bring them up because you don't know how to start the conversation. Or because you worry about having to describe your bowel movements, it's easier just not to mention them. If your symptoms are more vague in nature, such as fatigue or just feeling "out of it," they can be difficult to describe, too.

The celiac iceberg

Celiac disease experts often describe the disease in terms of an iceberg, a floating mass of ice with only its tip visible above water. Based on blood test screenings, it's estimated that around 1 percent of the American population has celiac disease. However, diagnosed cases are far fewer, closer to 0.17 percent.

The 0.17 percent is the tip of the iceberg, the visible part of the structure seen above water. These are the people who've been diagnosed with celiac disease — their blood tests are positive, biopsies confirm damage to their intestines, and they have symptoms associated with the disease.

The mass underneath the surface represents those who have celiac disease but don't know it. These might include people who have bothersome symptoms but who don't know the problem is celiac disease. They may never seek help, or they've received a wrong diagnosis.

The group below the waterline also includes those who aren't experiencing any symptoms that they could tie to celiac disease but who, if screened with genetic testing or blood tests, would have a positive result and whose biopsies would show intestinal damage. This group is sometimes referred to as having "silent" (asymptomatic) celiac disease. When they do get diagnosed, it's usually because a family member was diagnosed with celiac disease and they were encouraged to get tested even though they felt fine. Some estimates are that asymptomatic celiac disease is approximately seven times more common than is symptomatic celiac disease.

Finally, there are those individuals who have potential celiac disease — their genetic and blood tests are positive for celiac disease but a biopsy doesn't show any intestinal damage.

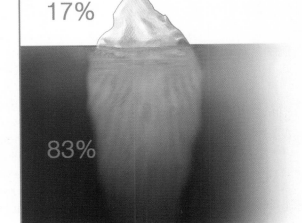

Diagnosed celiac disease — 17%

Undiagnosed celiac disease — 83%

© MFMER

MISSED OPPORTUNITIES Some people simply don't realize they have a problem. Their doctors may ask how they're feeling and they may say, "Just fine." Or when asked if they have any concerns with digestion or bowel movements, their response may be, "All's well." It's not that these individuals are being dishonest or trying to avoid their problems. They think they're fine — perhaps because their symptoms are mild or vague, they're so common, or they've lived with them so long. And it's not until after they're diagnosed with celiac disease that they realize what they considered normal really wasn't.

What's normal?

One of the first steps in seeking treatment for celiac disease is realizing that something isn't normal. If you've been experiencing symptoms for a long time — feeling bloated after meals, having constant headaches or frequent fatigue — you might not think anything is wrong. Because you've always had these symptoms, or you've had them for so long, they may seem normal.

Think about your typical day and ask yourself a few questions: Is that uncomfortable feeling you have after eating a passing phenomenon or a recurring theme? Are your mushy stools an occasional occurrence or is it something more? Do you generally feel tired or fatigued?

At one point or another, almost everyone experiences bouts of abdominal pain, diarrhea or excessive gas. These are common signs and symptoms that can result from eating too much or too fast, a viral infection, not exercising enough, or eating too many gas-producing foods. And certainly bowel habits vary widely. Some healthy people may have three bowel movements a week, while others may have three a day. And it's not uncommon for the frequency or the pattern of your bowel movements to change over time. And as you may well know, it's quite normal to feel tired or fatigued now and then.

However, if you regularly — not every time necessarily, but on a recurring basis — produce bowel movements that are loose and watery, or that look oily or greasy and float, talk to your doctor about it. Likewise, if your bowel movements are often accompanied by excessive or very malodorous gas — especially if your stools are mushy or watery — tell your doctor. The same is true for other symptoms. If they occur regularly, have them checked out.

Celiac disease damages your small intestine so that food can't be absorbed properly. This can lead to diarrhea and excessive gas. Persistent constipation, nausea or queasiness also warrant a medical appointment.

Even if it turns out that your symptoms aren't due to celiac disease, it's important to see your doctor. Don't accept diarrhea and mushy stools as normal because they're not. There's a reason behind them, and knowing why can help you address the problem.

This chart can help you determine if your bowel movements are normal. Almost everyone experiences each type of stool at one point or another. But if your bowel movements regularly produce stools similar to types 6 and 7, make an appointment with your doctor. Persistently loose or watery stools can be a sign of an underlying problem, such as celiac disease. Another feature of celiac disease is fatty stool (steatorrhea) — stool that's pale in color, bulky and often foul smelling. It may or may not have a greasy appearance. Steatorrhea results when fat passes through the small intestine unabsorbed and collects with the waste in your colon. Among children with celiac disease, some have very large stools that seem out of proportion for the size of the child.

Your stools can be an indicator of celiac disease

Bristol Stool Form Scale

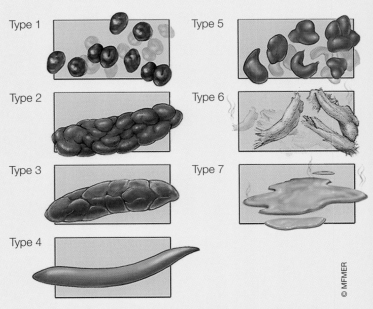

Type 1

Type 2

Type 3

Type 4

Type 5

Type 6

Type 7

© MFMER

Adapted from © Lewis SJ, et al. Stool form scale as a useful guide to intestinal transit time. *Scandinavian Journal of Gastroenterology.* 1997;32:921. Used with permission.

Taking stock of your situation

Sometimes it's difficult to tell how you're feeling from one day to the next. One way to get a more objective, big-picture look at your health is to keep track of your symptoms in a diary or on a calendar. Log anything that you feel isn't quite right, whether it be episodes of diarrhea, feeling overly tired or bloated, or having a headache. Mark down the date, time and the symptom. Try to provide as much detail as you can.

For example, if you had a bowel movement, was it soft and solid, loose and fragmented, or completely watery? Or when your stomach feels upset, does it feel bloated, achy, queasy or crampy? Also, when do these symptoms occur? Shortly after eating?

In addition, jot down what you ate at meals and if your symptoms seemed worse after eating certain foods. If you have time, it might also be beneficial to include what types of physical activity you engaged in, your emotional status, the medications you take, and when your period occurs if you're a woman. These extra details can help to provide a better context for the rest of your information and assist your doctor in making a diagnosis.

Keep the diary for at least two to four weeks. Over time, you may or may not see a pattern evolve. Most importantly, bring the information with you the next time you see your doctor so that you can have a more meaningful discussion with your doctor about what's bothering you and why.

Don't forget to evaluate your overall mood and the general quality of your life. How would you rate it on a scale from 1 to 5, with 1 being miserable and 5 being great? If you feel like you're consistently on the low end of the scale, tell your doctor about that, too. Sometimes, just not feeling well is a primary sign of an underlying problem, whether it be celiac disease or something else.

If keeping a journal sounds like too much work or it just isn't your thing, another approach that may help you assess your situation is to complete a symptoms questionnaire. The Celiac Disease Foundation (see page 274) has a symptoms checklist on its website that you can fill out to determine if you could be at risk of celiac disease and should see a doctor. You can get a copy of your responses to bring with you to your next doctor appointment.

Getting it right

A missed diagnosis isn't without its costs. People who've been interviewed before and after being diagnosed with celiac disease almost always say that their quality of life improved significantly once they finally learned what their problem was and they started on a gluten-free diet. In fact, not until after they start treatment and their symptoms disappear do some people realize how bothersome their symptoms were.

In addition to the daily annoyances, there are the potential long-term costs of leaving celiac disease undiagnosed and untreated — infertility, osteoporosis, other autoimmune disorders and gastrointestinal cancer.

If you think you might have celiac disease, or you're simply not sure, mention your concerns to your doctor. Don't dismiss your symptoms just because you may be uncomfortable talking about them, they seem to come and go, or they don't seem like a big deal. An honest conversation with your doctor can't hurt, and it may improve your health. Ask your doctor about testing for celiac disease and whether it might be a good idea for you. It's also important that you don't begin a gluten-free diet without first being tested for celiac disease. Chapter 11 will explain why.

Now, it may be that you've tried to talk to your doctor, or to several doctors, and no one seems to quite understand what you're trying to tell them. Or, perhaps, you've been given diagnoses and treatments that don't seem quite right or aren't working. If so, you may want to ask for a referral to a specialist, a gastroenterologist familiar with celiac disease. Don't give up on yourself or your health. Many people with celiac disease will tell you that it took many trips to the doctor and a lot of persistence before they finally learned what was wrong with them. At the end of this book, you'll find a list of resources that can help you find a celiac disease specialist or a support organization in your area.

The next chapter will guide you through the diagnostic process, and describe the different tests used to identify celiac disease. This information will also help you understand who should be screened for celiac disease and why.

CHAPTER FOUR

Getting the right diagnosis

You've thought about your symptoms, maybe even kept a diary for a few weeks, but you're still not sure what's going on. Truth is, your doctor can't determine if it's celiac disease based on symptoms alone. It can be easy to confuse the signs and symptoms of celiac disease with those of other conditions such as irritable bowel syndrome, chronic fatigue or other autoimmune disorders. And just because you may feel better after staying away from all foods that contain gluten doesn't mean you have celiac disease.

The good news is that there are reliable tests available to help distinguish celiac disease from other diseases and disorders. Testing for celiac disease is usually a two-step process: First, you undergo simple blood tests to check for certain antibodies that are commonly found in people with celiac disease. These screening tests can help detect celiac disease even if your symptoms are mild or you have no symptoms at all. But they don't provide a definitive diagnosis by themselves; they only identify people with a high probability of having celiac disease.

To confirm the results, you need an endoscopic biopsy. This is an outpatient procedure that allows your doctor to examine your small intestine and take several tiny tissue samples (biopsies) to check for damage to the lining of the intestine. If your blood tests are positive and the biopsy results indicate damage to the small intestine, then a diagnosis of celiac disease is made.

Before going through testing, however, there's an important caveat to remember. For test results to be accurate, it's essential that you're eating food that contains gluten. If you go on a gluten-free or low-gluten diet before being tested, your blood tests may come back normal even if you have celiac disease. If you receive a false-negative result, you may never know whether you really have celiac disease and if so, how much intestinal damage has occurred. If you're already on a gluten-free diet but are considering testing for celiac disease, your doctor may actually have you start eating gluten again. This is known as a gluten challenge (see page 72).

The thought of getting tested may seem intimidating or perhaps an unnecessary nuisance. You might be reluctant to go through with it, especially if you don't feel that bad or if you've started to feel better by avoiding gluten. On the other hand, if your symptoms are bothersome or have been occurring for a long time, knowing that a diagnosis can be obtained fairly easily may come as a relief.

An accurate diagnosis is in your best interest no matter where you're at. If test results show that you have celiac disease, a gluten-free diet will help you feel better quickly and help prevent long-term complications. If it turns out that you don't have celiac disease, you and your doctor are one step closer to finding other potential causes of your symptoms. And if you feel fine but you're being screened because you have close family members with celiac disease, negative test results can help you and your family rest assured that you're not in danger of celiac complications.

This chapter will help you learn who should get tested for celiac disease, what exactly is involved in the diagnostic process, which tests you'll need to undergo and any special issues that may crop up along the way. No single test can establish a diagnosis of celiac disease, but using several tests together allows your doctor to confidently determine if you have the disorder.

Who should be tested?

After reading the last couple of chapters, you may already have a good idea as to whether you should be tested for celiac disease based on your own experiences. However, the question of who should be checked for the disease has been a matter of considerable debate among doctors and scientists.

SCREEN EVERYONE? Sometimes the argument is made that everyone should be screened for celiac disease as a matter of course. This is based on the fact celiac disease is more common than previously thought, its signs and symptoms are so varied, and the way the disease presents itself seems to be continually changing. Furthermore, safe and effective treatment exists in the form of a gluten-free diet. However, mass screening poses several problems:

Benefits of treatment Issues associated with mass screening, including cost, must be balanced against the overall benefit to society. Many people identified in a mass screening as having celiac disease may have few if any symptoms. Current evidence suggests that people with asymptomatic or very mild celiac disease may not have the same risks as those whose symptoms are more prominent. Whether people who have no symptoms of celiac disease would reap enough benefit from a gluten-free diet to outweigh its cost and inconvenience is under debate.

Timing of screening Another challenge would be deciding when to screen an individual for celiac disease. Celiac disease can develop at any age, so would screening be best at birth? What if it developed later, in the adult years? How many times would a person need to be screened in order to receive a timely diagnosis? Screening would also have to occur during a time period where the disease can be diagnosed and treatment started before lasting damage has occurred. These are issues that add to the complexity of routine screening.

Accuracy of results Because the available screening tests for celiac disease aren't 100 percent accurate every time, it's possible that some people may test positive for celiac disease on a blood test but after a subsequent endoscopy and biopsy find out they don't have the disease. This is known as a false-positive, and it could mean a lot of needless invasive testing. Work is underway, however, to reduce the false-positive rate so this becomes less of an issue.

SCREEN SELECT INDIVIDUALS? Because of the current problems associated with screening everyone, the preferred approach at this point is to screen only individuals considered at high risk of celiac disease. What warrants high risk may depend on the doctor you're seeing but, in general, screening may be considered if you meet one or more of the following criteria:

Symptoms Signs and symptoms that may prompt testing include gastrointestinal symptoms, fatigue, skin rash, and tingling or numbness in the hands and feet. For more on symptoms see Chapter 2.

Unexplained abnormal lab test results This includes test results that reveal bone abnormalities, anemia or abnormal liver function, for which the cause is unknown.

Associated illnesses Celiac disease can express itself in literally hundreds of different ways. The presence of certain symptoms is often how the disease is first suspected. Sometimes, though, it's the development of other illnesses that eventually leads to a diagnosis of celiac disease (see opposite page).

Associated symptoms and conditions

There are many disorders known to be or believed to be associated with celiac disease. If you have one or more of the signs and symptoms below and you've been diagnosed with any of the diseases or conditions listed, your doctor may want to test you for celiac disease. This list isn't complete, but it provides an idea of symptoms or illnesses that may warrant screening:

Abdominal pain and bloating

Bulky or loose stools

Diarrhea

Nausea

Fatigue

Itchy skin rash (dermatitis herpetiformis)

Headaches

Heartburn

Tingling or numbness in hands and feet

Poor balance and coordination

Weight loss

Canker sores

Discolored teeth

Joint pain

Irritability or depression

Failure to thrive (children)

Delayed puberty and growth (children)

Anemia

Type 1 diabetes

Osteoporosis or osteopenia

Irritable bowel syndrome

Seizure disorder

Autoimmune hepatitis

Infertility

Thyroid disease

Sjögren's syndrome

Down syndrome

Microscopic colitis

Fibromyalgia

Rheumatoid arthritis

Lupus

Ataxia

Kidney disease

Liver disease

First-degree relative with celiac disease This may be a sibling, child or parent. Studies suggest that up to 20 percent of siblings and 10 percent of other first-degree relatives of individuals diagnosed with celiac disease also are affected. If you have a first-degree relative with celiac disease, mention this to your doctor. Even if you aren't experiencing symptoms you should be tested.

Blood tests

There are several blood tests that can serve as initial screening tests for celiac disease. They check for the presence of certain proteins called antibodies. When you have celiac disease, your immune system mistakenly identifies gluten as a foreign invader (an antigen). As a result, it produces antibodies that target gluten. In addition, your immune system also produces antibodies against some of your body's own proteins (autoantibodies). Elevated levels of these different types of antibodies in your bloodstream are generally a good indication of celiac disease.

A blood test for celiac disease is performed similar to other blood tests. A small sample of blood is drawn from a vein in your arm and then sent to a laboratory for analysis.

Although there are several blood tests available, some are more accurate and easier to analyze than others. For many people, the only blood test that may be necessary is the tissue transglutaminase antibody test. For a few people, however, other blood tests may be more appropriate.

The following blood tests may be used to test for celiac disease:

TISSUE TRANSGLUTAMINASE ANTIBODIES (TTG-IGA) This is the most common test used to identify celiac disease. Tissue transglutaminase (tTG) is a multifunctional enzyme that's found in everyone's small intestine. It's also involved in a special kind of processing (deamidation) of gliadin. Gliadin is a gluten particle (peptide) that triggers the immune response characteristic of celiac disease. The celiac immune response leads to the production of antibodies against regular gliadin peptides, deamidated gliadin peptides and the body's own tTG enzymes.

Testing for the presence of tTG antibodies is one of the simplest and most accurate ways to determine whether you might have celiac disease. People

Why it's important to double-check the results

Your body makes five families of antibodies — IgA, IgD, IgE, IgG and IgM. The most common antibody made by immune cells that line the digestive tract is IgA. A small percentage of people, however, don't produce any IgA, a condition known as IgA deficiency.

For reasons that aren't clear, people with celiac disease are more likely to have IgA deficiency. This is important when testing for celiac disease because if you're IgA deficient the results of blood tests to measure certain antibody levels may not be accurate. Test results may indicate you don't have celiac disease when in fact you really do.

This is why more than one test may be used to check for celiac disease or why a doctor may order a different test if the results of the initial test didn't produce the results he or she was expecting.

without celiac disease can have positive antibody test results. However, if you test strongly positive, chances are good you have celiac disease.

ENDOMYSIAL ANTIBODIES (EMA-IGA) Before the tTG test was developed, scientists discovered that people with celiac disease had high levels of antibodies directed at endomysial tissue, the thin tissue layer that covers muscle fibers in the intestine. A few years later, scientists discovered that tTG, which lives in endomysial tissue, was the real target of the antibodies. So the tTG and EMA tests essentially check for the same thing. The EMA test is time-consuming, expensive and more difficult, but it's very specific to celiac disease. Your doctor may request it if your tTG results are inconclusive or difficult to interpret. This test may also be used if a biopsy can't be performed.

TOTAL IGA Your body's immune system produces immune proteins (immunoglobulins) and different families of antibodies. Each family is indicated by letter — A, D, E, G and M. Most of the antibodies used to identify celiac disease come from the immunoglobulin A (IgA) family. Some come from the immunoglobulin G (IgG) family.

Both tTG-IgA and tTG-IgG tests are available, but the tests that measure the IgA class are more accurate and, therefore, generally the first choice. An IgG test may be used in specific circumstances when an IgA test may not produce a valid result, as in the case of IgA deficiency (see opposite page). An abnormal level of IgA alone doesn't indicate celiac disease. Additional testing is required to make a diagnosis.

DEAMIDATED GLIADIN PEPTIDE (DGP) Testing for antibodies to the tTG-processed version of gliadin (deamidated gliadin) is a fairly new test, but evidence suggests it may be helpful in detecting celiac disease in people who are IgA deficient. It may also be particularly useful for children under 2 years of age, in whom other tests may not be as good at identifying celiac disease (not as sensitive) as they are in older children and adults.

ANTI-GLIADIN ANTIBODIES (AGA) This test was one of the first blood tests to be developed for celiac disease. It measures levels of antibodies that directly target gliadin before it's been deamidated. The problem is that quite a few healthy people have increased levels of anti-gliadin antibodies, which means this test isn't very good at predicting who has celiac disease and who doesn't. It's generally not recommended as a method for identifying celiac disease because it's not as accurate.

No test for celiac disease is 100 percent accurate. If a blood test suggests you have celiac disease, typically the next step is an endoscopic biopsy of your small intestine. It could take a couple of weeks before the results of the blood test are back and before a biopsy can be performed. Don't change your diet until all testing is complete.

Before you proceed with tests for celiac disease, you may wish to contact your insurance company to see if they will cover the cost of the tests. Insurers will often cover diagnostic testing for celiac disease, such as antibody tests, if you have symptoms suggestive of the disease and if your doctor believes a diagnosis of celiac disease is possible. Testing may also be covered if you have a first-degree relative with celiac disease. Insurers may or may not cover initial testing for people who don't have symptoms related to celiac disease.

The same test also may be coded differently for insurance purposes and involve different charges. For example, testing for someone who is asymptomatic may not be billed in the same way that diagnostic tests for someone who has symptoms are billed. Since coverage varies based on insurers and the types of health insurance plans, your best bet is to contact your insurance company before testing so that you know if the tests will be paid for.

Biopsy

A diagnosis of celiac disease isn't complete until small samples (biopsies) of your intestinal lining have been examined under a microscope. Celiac disease causes small areas, or patches, on the lining of your small intestine to become inflamed. This typically occurs in the first part of the small intestine called the duodenum. Usually, your small intestine is lined with villi, tiny hairlike projections that help your intestine absorb nutrients. Celiac disease damages villi, sometimes to the point in which they become completely flattened out (villous atrophy) and are unable to absorb nutrients.

Generally, your doctor will request a biopsy after blood tests have come back positive for celiac disease. In some cases, though, even if your blood tests are negative, your doctor may proceed with a biopsy. An example is if the results of your blood tests are negative, but you have all of the classic signs and symptoms of celiac disease — diarrhea, weight loss, abdominal pain and fatty stools.

Endoscopy

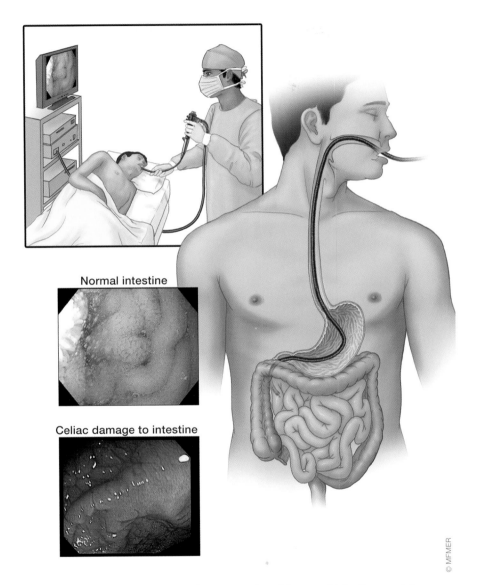

Normal intestine

Celiac damage to intestine

© MFMER

During an endoscopy procedure, tissue samples of the small intestine are taken while you're under sedation. The top photo shows how the lining of a healthy small intestine appears during an endoscopy procedure. You can see the tiny villi. The photo below it comes from the small intestine of an individual with celiac disease. The villi are flattened out, giving the lining the appearance of a tile floor.

Tissue samples of the upper intestine are obtained during an upper gastrointestinal endoscopy, a procedure that involves gently inserting a long, flexible tube (endoscope) down your throat and into your esophagus, stomach and upper small intestine while you're under sedation. Through this tube, your doctor inserts a camera to view your intestine and a small tool to collect tissue samples for analysis.

The tissue samples are sent to a specialist (pathologist) skilled at recognizing signs of disease in the samples. The pathologist will examine the tissue samples under a microscope and provide your doctor with a report. The report will indicate whether any damage is present and whether the damage is consistent with celiac disease.

Sometimes celiac disease is discovered by accident. An endoscopy may be performed for other reasons, and during the procedure the doctor may see patches of inflammation caused by celiac disease.

WHAT TO EXPECT DURING THE PROCEDURE An endoscopic biopsy might sound a little scary at first, but don't worry — there will be trained people there to help and guide you along every step of the way. Also, the procedure doesn't take that long — usually less than 15 minutes. It's generally recommended you avoid eating or drinking anything for several hours to ensure that your stomach is empty.

Before the procedure begins, you'll likely be given a sedative through a vein in an arm to help you relax and feel more comfortable. Although you might feel mentally alert, your reflexes, memory and judgment may be slow until the sedative wears off, which is why you can't drive home afterward. If you have a history of troubles with sedation, perhaps during a colonoscopy or dental work, or you take long-term benzodiazepines or opiate painkillers, mention this to your doctor beforehand. Instead of conscious sedation another form of sedation, such as general anesthesia, may be more appropriate.

In the exam room, you'll be lying on an exam table on your left side. Typically, monitors are attached to your body to allow your medical team to track your breathing, blood pressure and heart rate. To numb your throat, your doctor may spray an anesthetic in your mouth before the endoscope is inserted. You may be asked to swallow as the scope passes down your throat. Although you might feel some pressure in your throat, you shouldn't feel any pain.

As the endoscope goes through your esophagus, a tiny camera at the tip relays images to a video monitor in the exam room. Your doctor watches this monitor to look for abnormalities in your upper digestive tract and take pictures if necessary.

Celiac disease

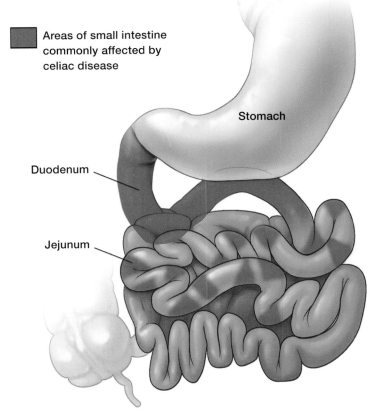

Areas of small intestine commonly affected by celiac disease

Stomach

Duodenum

Jejunum

© MFMER

Celiac disease often develops in patches. When tissue samples (biopsies) of the small intestine are taken, it's important they come from various locations, so as not to miss the disease.

When the endoscope reaches the small intestine, your doctor will insert a tiny surgical tool through the device to gently remove several tissue samples. Because celiac disease can affect some areas of the small intestine and not others, the American College of Gastroenterology guidelines recommend collecting at least four samples. If only one or two biopsies are taken, damaged areas may be missed and an inaccurate diagnosis made.

When your doctor has finished the exam, the endoscope is slowly removed through your mouth. You might stay in a recovery room for an hour or so, but you can go home pretty quickly after the procedure is over. Your throat may feel a little sore for a while and you might feel some temporary bloating or cramping, but these should go away in a day or two. If they don't, contact your doctor. Your doctor may meet with you after the exam to discuss visual findings. The biopsy results usually aren't ready for a few days after the procedure. You may receive them personally or in a written report.

Capsule endoscopy

Capsule endoscopy is a noninvasive way for your doctor to look at your small intestine. The technique uses a tiny wireless camera to take pictures of your entire small intestine. The camera sits inside a large vitamin-sized capsule that you swallow. As the capsule travels through your digestive tract, the camera takes thousands of pictures that are transmitted to a recorder.

Capsule endoscopy may be used if you're unable to undergo a regular endoscopy or if you have celiac disease that's complicated by ulcers or a mass in the small intestine. While the technique is very good at capturing extensive damage, it's not so good at detecting milder lesions.

Genetic tests

Genetic testing isn't a routine part of celiac disease testing, but in some cases it can be helpful in ruling out the illness. Thanks to advances in medicine, a lot is now known about the genetics of celiac disease and the importance of the human leukocyte antigen (HLA) genes in its development.

There are many different types of HLA genes. Those involved with celiac disease help convert information into code (encode) for substances that play a critical role in the functioning of your immune system, called DQ antigens.

Everyone carries two copies of the HLA-DQ genes. Almost all people with celiac disease carry specific forms that come together to encode proteins called HLA-DQ2 and HLA-DQ8. If you don't test positive for the HLA-DQ2 and HLA-DQ8 genes, it's unlikely that you have celiac disease. If you do carry one or both of these genetic markers, you could have celiac disease, but it isn't a guarantee. That's because the genes are also found in approximately 30 percent of the general population — people who don't have celiac disease. For this reason, the best use of genetic testing is to rule out celiac disease.

Unfortunately, some people are diagnosed with celiac disease based on genetic testing alone. Because they test positive for one or both of the associated genes, it's assumed they have celiac disease. They're told to follow a gluten-free diet when they don't actually have the disease. To know for sure if you have celiac disease, additional testing is needed.

WHY HAVE A GENETIC TEST? Genetic testing is a fairly simple and easy process, although it's fairly expensive. A blood sample is all that's required. Some labs will accept cheek swabs for genetic testing. You might consider genetic testing in the following circumstances:

You're in doubt Genetic testing can be useful when blood test results conflict with biopsy results. For example, if your blood tests are negative for celiac disease but your biopsy results show intestinal damage, genetic testing may help clarify the diagnosis.

You're at high risk People at high risk, such as those who have Down syndrome or Turner syndrome, may use genetic testing to rule out celiac disease so that they don't have to undergo other testing.

Family members of people with celiac disease may use genetic testing to determine if they're at risk of the disease. If someone in your immediate family is diagnosed with celiac disease, but you don't have symptoms and your blood tests are negative, genetic testing can determine if you need future testing.

If you test negative for the HLA-DQ2 and HLA-DQ8 genes, you don't have the disease and you're very unlikely to get it in the future. No more testing is needed. If you test positive, you could get the disease in the future, and you should consider continued periodic testing, especially if symptoms develop.

Because genes run in families, if a first-degree relative has celiac disease, the chances are pretty high — about 66 percent — that you also carry one of the genes associated with the disease. But you still only have a 1 in 6 chance of getting celiac disease.

You're already eating gluten-free Genetic testing may be helpful for someone who's already eating gluten-free but who hasn't been tested for celiac disease. After about a month of being gluten-free, antibody levels begin to return to normal and intestinal damage begins to heal, so blood and biopsy tests may come back negative even if you have celiac disease.

To get accurate results on antibody testing, it's necessary to reintroduce gluten into your diet for a few weeks before testing. This is called a gluten challenge. Before starting a gluten challenge, your doctor may recommend genetic testing. A negative result indicates that you don't have the genes associated with celiac disease and you don't need further testing for it. However, this doesn't mean you might not have non-celiac gluten sensitivity or another gluten-related problem (see Part 2 for more information).

If you test positive for the HLA-DQ2 and HLA-DQ8 genes, it doesn't mean that you have celiac disease. However, it does indicate that you should undergo further testing.

A gluten challenge

Increasingly, people are embarking on a gluten-free diet without first being diagnosed with celiac disease. Going gluten-free before testing won't harm you, but it can interfere with receiving an accurate diagnosis — knowing for certain that you have celiac disease.

For a celiac immune reaction to occur, you have to be eating gluten. If you're not eating gluten, your body has nothing to react to and the levels of antibodies and autoantibodies associated with celiac disease will eventually return to normal. Likewise, damage to your intestinal lining subsides. The villi grow back, and the lining's appearance may return to normal.

The amount of time it takes for the body to respond after eliminating gluten varies from one person to the next, but it can happen pretty quickly — often within a matter of weeks. Healing may occur especially quickly in children.

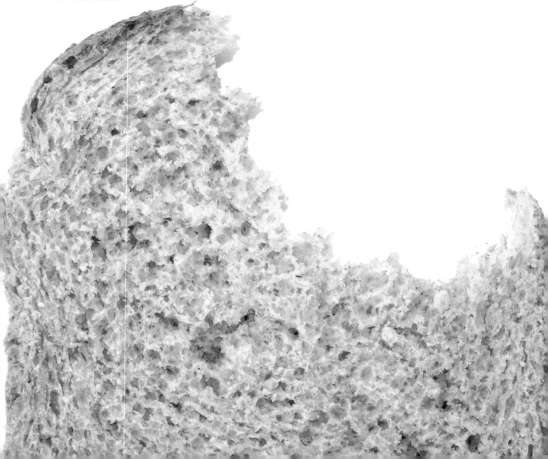

If you've been on a gluten-free diet for over a month, there's a good chance blood tests for celiac disease will come back normal or be inconclusive, and you won't know if you have the disease unless you have a biopsy, and even then the results may be questionable.

If your doctor suspects you may have celiac disease but your blood tests come back negative because you're already eating gluten-free, he or she may recommend that you undergo a gluten challenge to make sure you receive an accurate diagnosis.

WHAT'S INVOLVED? A gluten challenge involves reintroducing gluten into your diet for a certain period of time so that testing can determine whether your body's reacting to the gluten. Current guidelines issued by the American College of Gastroenterology (ACG) recommend that if you're on a gluten-free diet and your blood tests come back negative, you first undergo genetic testing to see if you carry one of the genes associated with celiac disease. If you test negative, you don't have celiac disease and no further testing is necessary.

If you do carry one of the genes, your doctor will likely recommend that you go back to a gluten-rich diet for several weeks. For a long time, this meant eating 10 grams of gluten — about four to five slices of wheat bread — every day for up to eight weeks. But this rate of gluten ingestion for such a long period of time caused many people to experience distressing symptoms that made it difficult to complete the challenge.

More recent evidence indicates that eating 3 grams of gluten — about two slices of wheat bread — every day for two weeks is enough to generate an antibody reaction in the majority of people with celiac disease.

Based on this evidence, the ACG recommends an initial two-week trial of eating gluten, followed by repeat blood tests and a biopsy. If your symptoms are tolerable during the gluten challenge, your doctor may opt to prolong the gluten challenge a few more weeks before testing to improve the accuracy of the diagnosis.

Once the gluten challenge is over and you've gotten your results back, you and your doctor can proceed with the next step. If you have celiac disease, this will involve returning to a gluten-free diet. If you don't have celiac disease, the two of you can explore other causes for your symptoms and perhaps more effective treatment for what's bothering you.

WHY DO IT? If you've started feeling better on a gluten-free diet, you may wonder why you should go back to eating gluten just to go through more tests. This is a valid question, and one that a lot of people ask.

The short answer is so you can get an accurate diagnosis — so that you know for certain that you have celiac disease. It's important to know what's

For children age 2 and older, the diagnostic process for celiac disease is roughly the same as for adults. For children younger than age 2, blood tests used in adults, such as the tTG and EMA tests, aren't as accurate. This is partly because infants and toddlers have been consuming gluten for a shorter amount of time, and it takes a while for antibodies to build up in the bloodstream.

For children younger than age 2, the preferred blood test is the newer DGP tests. Studies show that both DGP-IgA and DGP–IgG tests are very accurate in detecting celiac disease in younger children, close to 100 percent. DGP testing can also be useful in monitoring children for accidental sources of gluten ingestion once they begin a gluten-free diet.

If celiac disease runs in your family and you want your child tested, keep in mind that if the child hasn't eaten any gluten there's no point in doing any testing. A child can't develop celiac disease until he or she has eaten gluten.

Is a biopsy necessary? If you're a parent, watching your child undergo blood testing can be difficult enough. The possibility of your child having to go through an endoscopic biopsy might seem out of the question. However, biopsy of the upper intestine is still considered the gold standard for confirming a diagnosis of celiac disease in children and adults. Plus, it can serve as a reference to check for healing in biopsies that are performed later.

It might help to know that general anesthesia is used in most cases during a pediatric endoscopy, which means your child will be asleep during the procedure and likely won't remember a thing. In addition, a team of care providers will be monitoring your child before, during and after the procedure to make sure everything goes smoothly.

Still, the prospect of a biopsy can make any parent feel hesitant. Scientists have been trying to determine whether, based on blood test results, some children might be able to avoid the need for an intestinal biopsy. There's evidence that when tTG-IgA levels are very high — more than 10 times the normal limit — it's likely that a child who exhibits symptoms suggestive of celiac disease has damage to the intestinal lining.

The European Society for Pediatric Gastroenterology, Hepatology and Nutrition has suggested that a doctor may choose to make a diagnosis based on a child's symptoms and blood tests that indicate the presence of one of the specific HLA genes, very high levels of tTG and a positive EMA on a separate blood sample. It's also important that the child have a positive response to a gluten-free diet. Not everyone agrees with these guidelines and some studies have suggested that this method isn't as accurate as a biopsy. But it may provide an option for children who can't undergo an endoscopic biopsy.

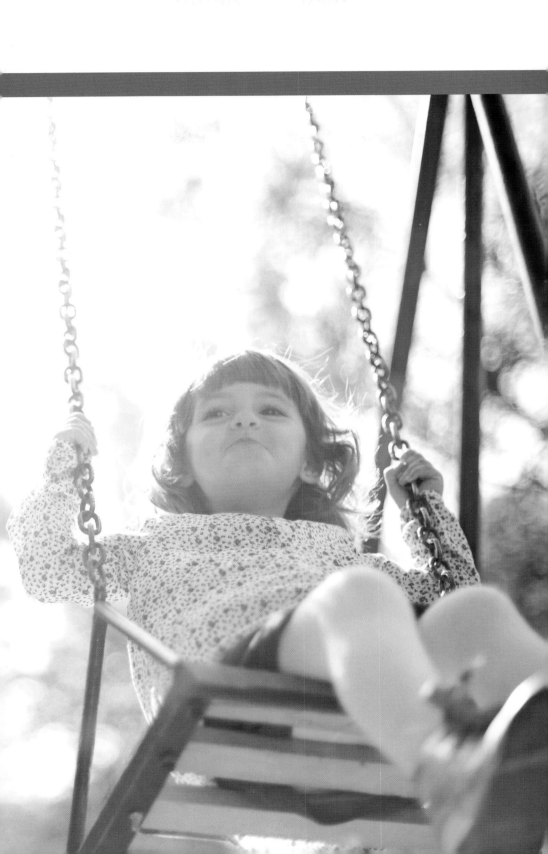

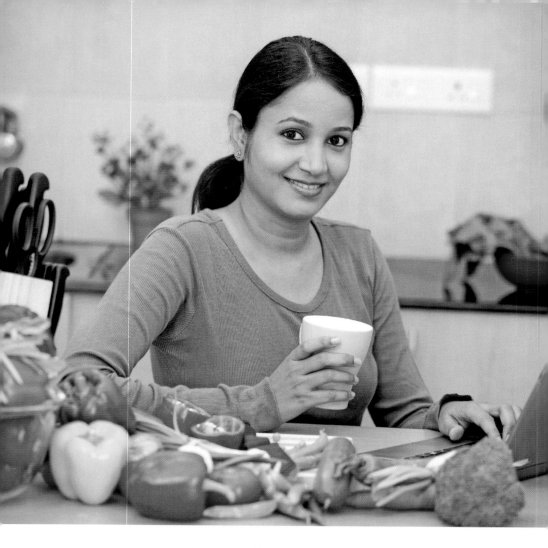

causing your symptoms because different diseases pose different risks of long-term complications. Because you're feeling better on a gluten-free diet, you may automatically assume that you have celiac disease. But it could be that you have irritable bowel syndrome or you're intolerant to something else in your diet.

Some people who feel dramatically better on a gluten-free diet are surprised to find out after undergoing a gluten challenge that they don't have celiac disease. These individuals may have non-celiac gluten sensitivity, or it may be that the symptoms they were experiencing are actually due to some other component of wheat. The symptoms got better on a gluten-free diet not because they're eating less gluten but because they're eating less of something else. This is discussed in more detail in Part 2 of this book.

Knowing for certain that you have celiac disease rather than something else can help you stick with a gluten-free diet because you know the risks involved if you cheat. And if you don't have celiac disease, it would be helpful to know what you do have. In addition, your family members may be able to avoid needless testing to see if they have celiac disease.

If you don't feel you can tolerate a gluten challenge, talk to your doctor about it. Depending on how long you've been gluten-free, your doctor may opt for an endoscopic biopsy to see if your intestinal lining still shows any signs of damage, since it can take some time for the small intestine to heal.

Sometimes, people elect to stay on a gluten-free diet without ever receiving a formal diagnosis. If this is the case, to avoid potential complications, you must be just as committed to a lifelong gluten-free diet as if you had been diagnosed with celiac disease.

Interpreting the results

Although it seems like the results of celiac disease testing should be pretty straightforward — either positive or negative — they aren't always clear-cut. Here are some common scenarios resulting from testing, along with what would likely happen next.

SYMPTOMS, POSITIVE BLOOD TESTS AND ABNORMAL BIOPSY If you have symptoms of celiac disease, your antibody blood tests are positive and your biopsy confirms intestinal damage, then you have a confirmed diagnosis of celiac disease. In this case, your doctor will talk to you about starting a gluten-free diet and ideally refer you to a dietitian experienced in treating celiac disease. Your doctor may ask you to be tested for any nutritional deficiencies — such as iron, folate, and vitamins B-12 and D — that may have resulted from the disease.

SYMPTOMS AND NEGATIVE BLOOD TESTS If you have symptoms of celiac disease but your blood tests are negative, it may be that you have selective IgA deficiency, in which case you should be tested with an IgG set of blood tests. Another possibility is that you're already on a gluten-free diet or eating small amounts of gluten, which can affect your blood test results. If this is the case, you may need to undergo a gluten challenge.

Sometimes, if your symptoms are highly suggestive of celiac disease, your doctor may proceed with an endoscopic biopsy to rule out the disease even if your blood tests are negative. It's also possible that the cause of your symptoms isn't celiac disease, but perhaps another nongluten-related disorder.

POSITIVE BLOOD TESTS AND NORMAL BIOPSY Occasionally, blood tests will come back positive for celiac disease but intestinal biopsies look normal.

The most common reason for this scenario is a false-positive blood test — a result suggesting celiac disease is present when it's not.

In this situation, your doctor may request a repeat blood test or ask for a second opinion on your biopsies. If this doesn't clarify the diagnosis, your doctor may ask you to eat gluten for several weeks and then repeat the biopsy, being sure to collect multiple samples from different sections of the intestine.

If your biopsy comes back normal, you may have what's referred to as potential celiac disease, meaning you might develop celiac disease in the future. At this point, switching to a gluten-free diet usually isn't necessary. However, your doctor may continue to monitor you with blood tests and have you alert him or her if you experience any new symptoms.

NO SYMPTOMS, POSITIVE BLOOD TEST AND ABNORMAL BIOPSY If you don't have any symptoms, but you were tested for celiac disease because someone in your family has it and the results came back positive, your doctor may tell you that you have asymptomatic, or "silent," celiac disease.

People with asymptomatic celiac disease generally tend to feel better after being gluten-free, even if they didn't think they had symptoms before being diagnosed. Your doctor may recommend getting tested for nutritional deficiencies, including a bone density test, to see if celiac disease has affected you in other ways that may not be obvious.

A ways to go

Despite all that's being done to identify people at high risk of celiac disease and screen for the disease, the fact remains most people who have it remain undiagnosed. There are many reasons for this, but two of the most common are the fact the disease can hide and that doctors often don't think of celiac disease when treating patients.

As mentioned in earlier chapters, symptoms of celiac disease can often be very subtle, and some people don't have symptoms at all. Celiac symptoms can also mimic other conditions, such as irritable bowel syndrome. In addition, people who may be bothered by cramps or loose stools after eating may not say anything to a doctor because they think what they're experiencing is normal.

By the same token, doctors often don't think of celiac disease when a patient complains of symptoms associated with the disease, so they don't test for it. This is partly because not that long ago the disease was rare and doctors didn't receive much training on it in medical school. In addition, the characteristics of the disease have changed. Celiac is no longer just a malabsorption

On occasion, some people are diagnosed with celiac disease when they really don't have the condition. How does this happen? Generally, an incorrect diagnosis results when not all of the diagnostic tests are performed. Most often, it occurs when biopsies taken during an endoscopic procedure reveal intestinal damage similar to celiac disease. But the biopsy findings aren't backed up by blood test results indicating the presence of specific antibodies associated with celiac disease. To make an accurate diagnosis, you need both.

An inaccurate diagnosis can also happen because certain medications and conditions can mimic the damage of celiac disease. Drugs that are associated with injury of the lining of the small intestine include the high blood pressure medication olmesartan (Benicar) and the immunosuppressive drug mycophenolate mofetil (CellCept), as well as nonsteroidal anti-inflammatory medications (NSAIDs). Other conditions that can produce damage similar to that of celiac disease include tropical sprue, immune deficiencies, bacterial overgrowth and Whipple's disease.

For people who receive an inaccurate diagnosis, their symptoms don't get better despite following a gluten-free diet. Further testing and examination reveal celiac disease is not the culprit.

Being told you have celiac disease when you really don't

disorder. It produces a wide range of symptoms, making it more difficult to identify. A big challenge currently facing doctors and researchers is uncovering the disease in the many people who have it before these individuals develop serious complications.

In the next few chapters, you'll learn more about coping with a new diagnosis of celiac disease and finding effective ways to make the transition to a gluten-free lifestyle.

CHAPTER FIVE

Coming to terms with your condition

When you receive a diagnosis of celiac disease, it can evoke a variety of emotions — relief at finally knowing the source of your symptoms, disbelief that you have a disease that you know little about, uncertainty as to how you'll manage a gluten-free lifestyle, and perhaps even deep sadness in learning that celiac disease is a permanent, lifelong condition that requires a pretty drastic lifestyle change.

Diagnosis of a lifelong illness is never easy. It often requires a certain amount of adjustment — physically, mentally and emotionally — before you become accustomed to a new way of living. Celiac disease is no different.

Treatment involves eliminating all gluten from your diet, which means avoiding all foods containing wheat, barley or rye, and oats, too, because oats are easily contaminated by the other three. These types of foods constitute a huge part of the American diet. Plus, ingredients that contain gluten are in many processed foods. Not being able to eat these foods is a real loss for many people. It's not uncommon to feel angry at your diagnosis, or to deny or hide from it in the hopes that it will all just go away.

It's OK to take some time to process all the information that's been given to you. It's a lot to absorb. But you should know that for most people with celiac disease, the benefits of eating gluten-free outweigh the costs. While it's important not to repress feelings of sadness, anger or resentment that might arise, it's also important to not get stuck in them. Using the support of those around you, as well as the information in this and other chapters, you can formulate a plan to move your life forward in a healthy and meaningful way.

Furthermore, you don't have to go it alone. Ideally, after your diagnosis, you'll be connected to a dietitian experienced with celiac disease who can help you transition effectively to a gluten-free lifestyle and offer continued advice as needed. There are also a growing number of support groups where you can meet and talk with other people who are in similar situations. Even if you don't have access to a local source of support, there's a strong support community online that can help you navigate the complexities of living gluten-free.

This chapter will help you understand the benefits and challenges of treating celiac disease, discuss the importance of working with an experienced dietitian, and offer tips on getting the most from your support community. Although you may feel overwhelmed at first, there's no reason why you soon can't be handling your new lifestyle like a pro.

Your feelings are normal

Often, one of the first reactions to a diagnosis of celiac disease is disbelief — how can this be happening to me or how can something as familiar and comforting as pasta or bread be the cause of what's hurting me? Disbelief may give way to feelings of frustration and anger. You might feel as if your life will never be the same or that it will be ruined forever because you won't be able to eat the things you like anymore.

You might also feel somewhat lost. Food is an important part of everyday life and culture. It helps us celebrate birthdays and holidays, weddings, and rites of passage. It often plays a central role in family get-togethers and outings with friends. Having to make major changes in the way you eat can make you feel like you're losing a big part of your personal identity or that you won't be able to travel or socialize in the same ways you did before. You might feel sad, anxious or lonely. Some people feel guilty as well, as if they've brought the illness on themselves. Or they tell themselves if they had done something differently, all of this wouldn't have happened.

Just the opposite, for people who've been battling symptoms for a long time without knowing what was wrong, a diagnosis of celiac disease brings incredible relief to finally know the root of the problem. If this is you, at last you have an accurate diagnosis and effective treatment to boot. However, it's not uncommon to lose some of that joy as you get into the nuts and bolts of learning how to eat gluten-free.

ANGIE'S STORY

My gluten journey started unexpectedly when my oldest sister went to see her dermatologist because of a rash on her elbow that wouldn't go away. Her doctor knew right away she had dermatitis herpetiformis and sent her to a specialist who tested her for celiac disease. The tests came back positive.

After my sister told our family she had celiac disease, two of my sisters were tested and the results were negative. Initially, I wasn't going to get tested. I didn't want to change what I ate or the way I shopped for groceries. My sister reassured me that it wasn't so bad, and eventually she talked me into getting tested. When I learned I had celiac disease, I was upset. I didn't feel sick, and I didn't want to change the way I was living.

Looking back, I realize I did have symptoms but I thought they were normal for me. My dentist told me my tooth enamel was wearing away. I was also iron deficient, and I was bothered by fatigue, heartburn, bloating and diarrhea. I didn't experience these symptoms every day, but when I would eat out or eat certain foods I would have to run to the bathroom.

After my diagnosis, my husband and teenage daughter didn't think having celiac disease was such a big deal. But as I told them more about it, they realized how important it was for me to make a change to my diet.

I'm adjusting well to a gluten-free lifestyle. I definitely can tell that I feel better! I don't have bloating or diarrhea like I used to. I don't feel as fatigued as I was before. I do still have heartburn, but it's controlled with medication. I'm not tempted by foods that contain gluten because I know I can't have them, and I feel I'm eating healthier by avoiding them. I had a blood test again six months after my diagnosis, and my numbers were very close to normal.

I must admit having celiac disease isn't always easy. It's difficult to participate in potluck meals because I don't know if the dishes contain gluten. Gluten-free foods are more expensive. Plus, my family doesn't like the gluten-free diet, so I often cook differently for myself.

At first it was overwhelming, but it's gotten easier. I've learned of so many people who also are eating gluten-free, and many restaurants now offer a gluten-free menu. Grocery stores have more gluten-free foods as well. I remind myself that foods such as vegetables, fruits and meats are naturally gluten-free, so it's not as if I'm totally limited.

I would strongly suggest anyone who thinks he or she might have a problem with gluten get tested. It was frightening for me because I didn't want to change my diet and I didn't want to put any extra effort into it. But it was definitely worth it. If you've just been diagnosed, try not to get too overwhelmed. Help is out there, and soon you'll feel so much better!

For some people, their initial reaction is neither anger nor relief but more a feeling of shock. They feel overwhelmed. There's so much to absorb it can be difficult to take it all in at once. They feel lost, not sure where or how to begin.

All of these responses are very normal. And it's totally fine to work through one set of feelings at a time. With time and a little patience, most people are able to adapt to their new circumstances. After the initial reaction wears off, they move in to an acceptance and motivational phase. They accept what's been handed to them, learn what they need to do to get healthy, and go to work.

At the moment, perhaps, it may not feel as if you'll ever adjust, but know that you will learn how to live gluten-free. And you'll come to find out that you really can live and eat well without gluten.

Consider the positives

At first you may feel nowhere near lucky — quite the opposite, perhaps — that the treatment for your illness involves a major shift in your diet. You know it will likely mean the permanent loss of some of your favorite foods, or a change in how they're made. However, it may be helpful to also consider some of the positive aspects of your illness.

NO SURGERY OR MEDICATIONS ARE NECESSARY Treatment for many illnesses often requires that you take medication daily or that you undergo an invasive surgical procedure to fix the problem. These kinds of treatments can have bothersome side effects or require a fairly extensive recovery period after the procedure. Sometimes, it can take a lot of tinkering to fine-tune treatment before its benefits outweigh the side effects or possible complications.

With a gluten-free diet, you experience benefits right away. There are generally no pills to take — unless you happen to need supplements for a nutritional deficiency — and no treatment procedures to go through. The diet usually starts working within a matter of days and with no real side effects. Most people with celiac disease feel much better within a few weeks. They have more energy and vitality, and they're experiencing far fewer painful or bothersome symptoms.

YOU'RE IN CHARGE Aside from working with a dietitian and seeing your doctor for regular checkups, treatment for celiac disease is largely do-it-yourself. And in the long run, you may find that there's a certain amount of comfort knowing that you're in control of your treatment and that you can heal your body on your own.

There's no doubt it can be a challenge at first. Determining what's gluten-free and what's not can be confusing and overwhelming, cleaning out your kitchen can be a hassle, and learning how to protect yourself against accidental gluten ingestion can be exhausting. But eventually, you may find that life without gluten is what it is — part of your being, part of who you are — and the process becomes easier to handle and accept.

YOU HAVE MORE OPTIONS In many ways, the popularity of gluten-free eating has been a boon for people with celiac disease. The food industry has quickly responded to the growing demand for gluten-free foods, stocking grocery shelves with more gluten-free products.

The quality of gluten-free foods also is improving as chefs and manufacturers find ways to make dishes tastier and more satisfying. Restaurants increasingly offer gluten-free foods on their menus, and bakeries have popped up solely to supply the demand for gluten-free baked goods. A variety of gluten-free cookbooks also are available at many bookstores, and recipes are only a click away on the Internet.

Even if the trendiness wears off, the increase in awareness and access to gluten-free foods will likely continue, to your benefit.

Seek out a dietitian

After learning that you have celiac disease, you may wonder what's next. One of the most important first steps you can take toward making a successful transition to a gluten-free lifestyle is to see a registered dietitian.

A registered dietitian is an expert in food and nutrition who has met specific educational and professional requirements. A dietitian's job is to translate the medical jargon of nutrition into practical solutions for your life.

A qualified dietitian experienced in working with celiac disease can give you the help and support you need as you learn how to eat gluten-free. Ideally, your doctor will refer you to a dietitian after informing you that you have celiac disease. If this doesn't happen, find a qualified dietitian yourself. You can ask your doctor for a referral, or you can search online for a registered dietitian near you who specializes in celiac disease or gluten disorders through the Academy of Nutrition and Dietetics' website (see page 274).

Medical insurance will often cover a certain number of visits with a dietitian, but some insurance providers may require a referral from your doctor. Make sure to check with your insurance company to see what's required.

WHAT TO EXPECT When you meet with a dietitian, he or she likely will talk with you about a number of different aspects about your life. The conversation may begin with an overview of your current health, including how you're feeling and any symptoms you may be experiencing. He or she may ask about your weight to determine if you're underweight, overweight or at a healthy weight. He or she may also ask you about prescription medications or supplements you take. You may discuss your general quality of life, including your overall mood, how physically active you are and how involved you are in social activities.

The conversation will likely include additional information about celiac disease and gluten. The two of you may discuss your current diet — your eating habits, who prepares your meals, where you often eat, the types of foods you like — and determine which foods you can still eat and which you will need to change. If someone else, such as your spouse, prepares most of your meals, it's important that he or she come with you to your appointment.

Finally, meeting with a dietitian is a lot like having your own personal cheerleader or motivator. He or she can help you set goals and prepare you for the changes ahead. After your first meeting, your dietitian may schedule a follow-up visit to make sure you're on track and doing well with your new eating plan.

WHAT YOU'LL LEARN After your dietitian has performed a thorough review of your health and your eating habits, he or she will help you create a personalized eating plan that keeps you away from gluten and that fits your lifestyle and preferences. The two of you will discuss a number of strategies that can be helpful to you as you transition to a gluten-free diet. This information is discussed in detail in Part 3 of this book, but here's an overview.

How to create a healthy meal plan A dietitian can direct you to meals that you can prepare and the ingredients that you'll need to make them. The best approach is to start simple and expand your menu when you feel more comfortable about what foods and food ingredients do and do not contain gluten.

Keep in mind that just because you eat food that's labeled "gluten-free" doesn't mean it's healthy. A dietitian can help you come up with a meal plan that provides you with the essential nutrients your body needs. A healthy, gluten-free diet looks a lot like a regular balanced diet. It generally consists of fruits and vegetables; unprocessed lean meats; dairy products or milk alternatives; potatoes, rice and other gluten-free grains.

A dietitian can also refer you to cookbooks and recipes that can help you prepare gluten-free meals that your whole family can enjoy.

How to read labels A food doesn't need to be labeled gluten-free for it to be safe to eat. One way to know if a food contains gluten is to check the ingredient list. A dietitian will teach you what to look for to know if there's gluten in the product. If you see ingredients such as flour, semolina, durum, malt, bulgur and brewer's yeast, you'll know it's not for you.

What gluten-free labels mean A surprising number of products that normally contain plenty of gluten today are labeled "gluten-free," including bread, pasta and cereal. Are they really completely free of gluten? You'll learn what gluten-free claims and logos mean.

How to keep your kitchen safe A dietitian will help you understand the dangers of cross-contamination in the kitchen and how to maintain a home that's safe from gluten. He or she will explain how to thoroughly clean all of your cooking utensils and items that you may want to designate as your own and not share with others in the family.

How to avoid accidents A common reason people continue to feel poorly after starting a gluten-free diet is because they're still ingesting gluten and they don't know it. Your dietitian can help you identify and eliminate hidden sources of gluten.

Find support

At first you might feel like you're facing this new phase of your life on your own, but you're not. You might be surprised at how supportive family and friends can be, especially once they know how much better you'll feel not eating gluten and how important it is for your health. And if you make it an adventure, some of them may even be willing to tag along and try new foods with you. For example, you might come up with your own "Gluten-Free Food Review" where you and your family and friends rate different foods and make notes on which ones are keepers and which ones not so much.

Sharing a sense of humor is a great way to cope with the challenges of your new diet. Laughing with family and friends can ease the disappointment of a flopped recipe or less than ideal restaurant experience. And it can help you build up resilience and give you the strength you need to handle the next hurdle.

Your doctor and your dietitian also can be great sources of support. Ideally, you should have regular follow-ups with them, and they can answer any questions that you might have. They may also be able to connect you with people familiar with local resources, such as restaurants that have gluten-free menus or bakeries with gluten-free goods.

Another resource you might find helpful is a support group for people with celiac disease. People who've been living gluten-free for a while are often

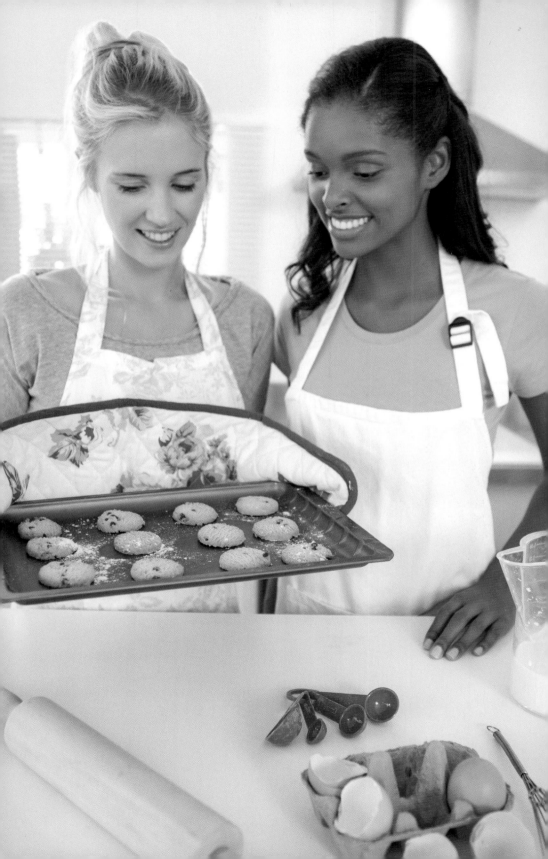

Don't be fooled by all that you hear and read

As you may know, celiac disease and gluten are hot topics these days. A simple search on the Internet using terms such as *celiac* or *gluten-free* will yield millions of results. Although it's great that there's so much interest, it's also important to sift through what you find so that you have accurate and reliable information you can depend on. Otherwise, you may end up with a lot of information but little real knowledge of celiac disease. This can result in confusion and frustration and even misinformation about how to avoid gluten.

Beware of advice from well-meaning people that conflicts with what you've learned from your doctor or dietitian. Health food stores and alternative health practitioners, such as chiropractors, provide useful services for some conditions, but there's little they can offer when it comes to celiac disease. High-priced gluten-free vitamins or chiropractic adjustments haven't been studied or proved helpful. The only proven way to heal celiac disease is to follow a gluten-free diet.

Make sure the information you're finding or the products you're purchasing are from reputable sources. The unfortunate truth is that not everyone has your best interest at heart. With all of the attention gluten is receiving, there are plenty of people hoping to cash in on the gluten-free craze by marketing "natural" products — from vitamins to special supplements to alternative treatments — that claim to treat celiac disease and other gluten disorders. Most products you can buy over-the-counter or online that claim to cut the amount of gluten in food or ease its digestion haven't been tested in good scientific studies to see if they work.

Use your good judgment. Don't spend money on treatments that aren't likely to help. If you're considering an alternative treatment or supplement, run it past your doctor or dietitian before you make the purchase. He or she can help you decide whether it's a reasonable option.

At the back of this book, you'll find a list of reliable resources to help you discover more about celiac disease, gluten-free living and celiac support organizations (see pages 274 and 275).

willing to share their hard-earned experience and knowledge and direct you to the best stores for gluten-free items or the tastiest gluten-free pizzas. Your doctor or dietitian might know of a support group near you, or you can search online. You can find a list of local chapters of the Celiac Support Association on its website (see page 274), or do an Internet search of celiac disease support groups in your area.

Maintain perspective

Remember that it's perfectly normal to experience a lot of different emotions after being diagnosed with celiac disease. It marks a major turning point, and the changes you're about to make will be lifelong. It takes time to process such a big transition.

At the same time, keep in mind that the journey you're about to embark on will almost certainly make you feel better and will eliminate all or at least most of the symptoms you've been experiencing.

And because it is a journey, it's OK to pause and make a plan, together with your family and your medical team, as to how you'll proceed. It might even help, in practical terms, to keep a notebook or a file folder where you can keep information that may help you along the way.

Take your journey one step at a time, and soon you'll be surprised at how far you've come. At first, it may seem like your new diet is very restrictive, but over time you'll learn about more foods you can eat that are both gluten-free and tasty. And along the way, you may meet new friends following a similar path as you. Together you can embark on some enjoyable journeys.

In the next chapter, you'll learn more about the management of celiac disease — how your doctor will monitor your condition to make sure your small intestine is healing and that you aren't at risk of complications.

CHAPTER SIX

Managing celiac disease

An amazing thing about the human gut is its ability to fix itself. Once you stop eating gluten, your immune system stops attacking your small intestine. The inflammation subsides, and the tiny villi that line the intestine begin to grow back. In many cases, though not in all, the intestine returns completely to normal. As this happens, other symptoms you may be having will disappear as well. Within a few weeks, sometimes even a few days, most people begin to feel better.

Successful management of celiac disease is about making sure your small intestine has the opportunity to heal. This is done by completely eliminating gluten from your diet. Management is also about watching out for other problems you may be experiencing because of your disease and making sure they're properly treated. This includes conditions such as nutrient deficiencies, lactose intolerance, anemia or osteoporosis.

When you're diagnosed with celiac disease, your doctor may perform several tests to see if you have any nutrient deficiencies, such as low levels of iron, folic acid, or vitamins D and B-12. Inadequate nutrient levels can develop when intestinal damage prevents your body from digesting your food as it should and absorbing key nutrients.

It's often recommended that people newly diagnosed with celiac disease take a daily multivitamin, at least for the first few months, to help treat conditions caused by low nutrient levels. Later in this chapter, you'll read more about vitamin and mineral supplements you may need.

After your diagnosis, your doctor will likely want to see you in a few months for a follow-up visit. You may also meet again with a dietitian to review your diet plan and review any questions or concerns you might have.

This chapter will help you understand what you can expect as you start off on your gluten-free journey, how your doctor and dietitian can help, and new treatments that might be on the horizon.

What to expect

Treatment for celiac disease centers around eliminating gluten from your diet. How to do this is discussed in great detail in Part 3 of this book, where you'll find everything you need to know about eating gluten-free.

After you begin your new diet, a number of changes may occur, virtually all of them positive. In general, following a gluten-free diet should:

⁑ Heal intestinal damage
⁑ Prevent new damage from occurring
⁑ Make you feel better
⁑ Eliminate all or most of your symptoms
⁑ Correct vitamin and mineral deficiencies
⁑ Heal skin rashes caused by dermatitis herpetiformis
⁑ Prevent long-term complications

Once you stop eating foods that contain gluten, your small intestine begins to repair itself. However, complete healing may take months or sometimes even years. The time it takes for your body to heal depends on a number of factors. One of them is age. Healing typically is more complete and rapid in children than it is in adults, but even in children, healing may not occur completely. Other factors include how long you've had the disease, how much damage it's caused, your overall health and how well you're able to avoid gluten.

YOUR SYMPTOMS Most people with celiac disease — about 70 percent — feel much better within a couple of weeks of eliminating gluten from their diets. In fact, some people begin to feel better within just 48 hours of not eating gluten. Signs and symptoms such as bloating, gas, diarrhea and abdominal pain go away fairly quickly when there's no gluten to irritate your gut. You may also find you have fewer headaches and more energy.

Evidence suggests that the villi in your intestine start to grow back within a few weeks of not being exposed to gluten, but it can take from a few months to several years for the intestinal lining to regain a healthy appearance and full function. The more severe the damage, the longer it usually takes to heal. But even in cases of severe, long-standing celiac disease, a gluten-free diet can lead to complete or almost-complete healing. The earlier the disease is diagnosed and the better you are at eliminating gluten from your diet, the better your chances are for complete healing.

Typically, symptoms improve faster than the intestinal lining does. Why this happens isn't quite clear. In general, the first portion of small intestine (duodenum) is the most severely affected because it receives the greatest amount of gluten exposure. The damage tends to lessen as the intestine leads into the colon. After you begin a gluten-free diet, the lower part of the small intestine generally recovers faster than the duodenum.

Recovery of the lower intestine allows for increased absorption of nutrients even while the duodenum is still healing. A better functioning small intestine improves signs and symptoms such as diarrhea, gas and bloating. Greater absorption of nutrients causes your body's vitamin and mineral levels to return to normal, so you feel less tired and more energetic.

YOUR WEIGHT For many people with celiac disease, a gluten-free diet helps to normalize their body weight. People who were underweight often gain weight on a gluten-free diet. Some people who were overweight lose weight because they're eating a more healthy diet. Others experience no changes in body weight after starting a gluten-free diet.

Be prepared for the possibility that you might gain weight on a gluten-free diet. It's not uncommon for people who are unable to properly absorb food, as happens with celiac disease, to develop an internal drive to eat more to make up for the loss of calories. This extends the set-point at which they feel satisfied. After starting a gluten-free diet, the set-point may still be abnormally high. Combined with the fact that as the intestine heals and you absorb more of the nutrients and ingredients in the food you eat, the result can be excessive weight gain.

Remember that just because a food is gluten-free doesn't mean it's healthy. Some prepackaged gluten-free foods are higher in fat, sugar and calories than regular versions.

To help prevent unwanted weight gain, you want to follow a balanced gluten-free diet. This means eating plenty of fresh fruits and vegetables, lean protein and dairy products, and whole, gluten-free grains. It also means limiting prepared or processed foods. A dietitian can help you develop a personalized eating plan that can help you maintain a healthy weight.

Exercising regularly also can help. As you begin to feel less fatigued and more energetic, consider adding a regular exercise routine to your weekly schedule. Exercise is important not just for maintaining a healthy weight. It can also help strengthen your bones, relieve feelings of stress and anxiety and help you feel better all around.

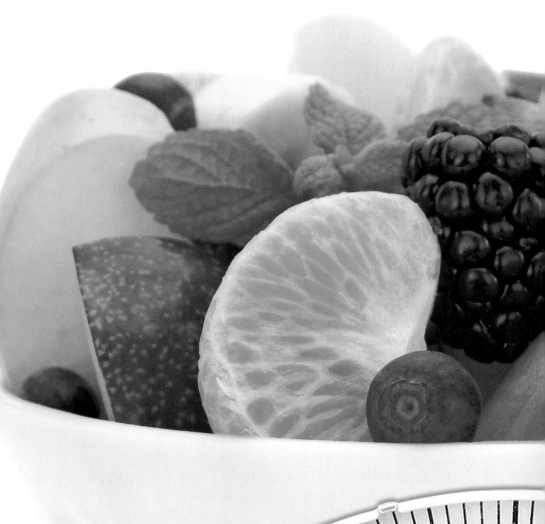
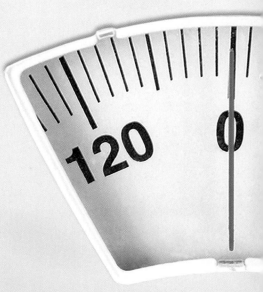

OTHER CONDITIONS Once you stop eating gluten, your body should begin to operate normally again. Many of the complications associated with celiac disease — such as lactose intolerance, infertility and reduced bone density — should improve.

Lactose intolerance People with celiac disease often experience lactose intolerance due to intestinal damage caused by celiac disease. When the small intestine is inflamed, it's not able to digest the natural sugar (lactose) in dairy products. In addition to eliminating gluten from your diet, you may also need to avoid certain dairy products for a period of time.

A simple test can help you determine if you still have trouble with dairy after avoiding it for six months or so. Drink a glass of milk in the morning on an empty stomach. If you don't experience any symptoms, then it's likely your ability to digest lactose has been restored. If symptoms of lactose intolerance persist, it may be a sign that you still have intestinal damage and you need to wait longer before trying to consume dairy products high in lactose.

Sometimes, celiac disease and lactose intolerance can exist separately. The intolerance continues after the small intestine is healed. In this case, you may need to limit certain dairy products the rest of your life, as well as avoid gluten.

Should I take probiotics?

Some evidence suggests that consuming probiotics as part of a gluten-free diet may promote intestinal healing in people with celiac disease. Probiotics is the name for healthy bacteria — bacteria that's considered "good" for digestion. Probiotics are commonly found in foods such as yogurt and kefir, a drink similar to yogurt. Probiotics also are sold as supplements.

Ask your doctor or a dietitian about adding probiotic foods or supplements to your diet. As long as they're gluten-free and they don't bother you, there's likely no harm in including them in your diet. However, if after a month or so you don't feel the supplement is providing any benefit it probably makes little sense to keep taking it.

Fertility Some people with celiac disease experience problems that affect their reproductive systems and their fertility. As you begin to absorb key nutrients, reproductive functions that may have been off-kilter should return to normal. If you're a woman and you were experiencing irregular menstrual cycles, your periods will probably become more regular.

Among couples experiencing problems with infertility, hormonal and reproductive functions often return to normal once a gluten-free diet is started. This is true for both women and men with celiac disease. Once women with celiac disease eliminate gluten from their diets, risk of miscarriage also is reduced.

This may be a good opportunity to talk to your doctor about family planning or revisit options for birth control, especially if you were relying on infertility as a method of family planning. Occasionally surprises can occur, even later in a woman's reproductive life.

Bone health It's not uncommon for people with celiac disease to have weakened bones. Celiac disease can affect absorption of calcium and vitamin D. Low levels of these important nutrients can weaken your bone structure and increase your risk of osteoporosis.

Once gluten is eliminated from your diet, your bone density should improve, reducing your risk of bone fracture. However, your doctor or a dietitian may recommend calcium and vitamin D supplements to help make up for any deficiencies. Exercising regularly also can help build bone and strengthen the muscles and ligaments that help protect bone.

Your doctor will likely want you to get screened for osteoporosis at least once after being diagnosed with celiac disease. Often the screening occurs shortly after the diagnosis is made. Depending on the results, part of your treatment plan may include medications such as bisphosphonates to increase bone density.

Additional issues Other problems associated with celiac disease such as joint pain, tingling and numbness in your hands and feet (peripheral neuropathy) and skin rash (dermatitis herpetiformis) may take longer to go away after beginning a gluten-free diet.

With peripheral neuropathy, it can sometimes take a couple of years to achieve maximum recovery. You might see reduced numbness or tingling in your arms first and then your legs, with the toes being the last to recover.

If you lived with celiac disease for many years before it was diagnosed, you might find that recovery may not always be complete. Your body may heal, but it may never return to normal. People with long-standing celiac disease may experience lasting complications that require continued treatment.

For example, some people who've developed difficulties with balance and walking (ataxia) as a result of celiac disease often find their symptoms improve on a gluten-free diet, but they don't disappear completely. In addition, while a gluten-free diet will treat celiac disease, it may not improve other autoimmune diseases such as type 1 diabetes or autoimmune thyroid disease. Management of your condition may also include ongoing monitoring of other disorders.

Key nutrients

Because celiac disease can interfere with your body's ability to absorb key nutrients from the food you eat, your doctor will likely want to perform tests to see if you have any vitamin or mineral deficiencies. This type of testing often occurs at the same time the disease is diagnosed. Or your doctor may request the tests shortly after you've been diagnosed. Your dietitian's assessment also can play an important role in diagnosing nutritional deficiencies.

Because your body needs certain levels of nutrients for good health and to function properly, your doctor and a dietitian will want to identify and treat any vitamin and mineral deficiencies. Some of the most common vitamins and minerals a doctor or dietitian will assess include iron, calcium, vitamin D, folic acid and vitamin B-12. Sometimes celiac disease can cause deficiencies of thiamine, copper, magnesium, zinc, selenium and vitamin B-6 as well.

Once you eliminate gluten from your diet and your small intestine begins to heal, most of these nutrient problems should resolve on their own. However,

Managing celiac disease in children

With early diagnosis and prompt treatment, growth and development quickly return to normal in children with celiac disease. In general, the younger a person is when beginning a gluten-free diet, the more likely the body will recover completely.

Because bones grow rapidly in childhood, bone density generally returns to normal levels soon after gluten is removed. If puberty hasn't hit yet, children who were shorter than their peers generally experience a growth spurt and are likely to reach their full adult potential.

In adolescents, a gluten-free diet should restore normal hormone cycles. Girls who've reached the age of puberty may soon experience menstrual cycles after gluten is removed, or experience them at the normal time. If menstruation has already begun, periods should even out and become more regular. Some evidence suggests that a gluten-free diet also helps with depression, which can be more common in teens with celiac disease than in adults with the disease.

Following a gluten-free diet can be a challenge for children and teens, especially if they feel they're not fitting in. Having a good support system in place can help. Chapter 18 has more information on helping kids live gluten-free.

especially in the beginning, you may need to take a daily multivitamin or a mineral supplement. Because gluten-free grains and cereals often aren't fortified or enriched with extra vitamins and minerals, your doctor or dietitian may recommend that you continue to take a multivitamin or mineral supplement even after the disease has gone into remission. Mineral supplementation is especially important for women of childbearing age.

CALCIUM AND VITAMIN D Calcium and vitamin D are important for everyone, but especially so for people who have celiac disease. Since celiac disease can increase your risk of bone disease, it's important that you're getting adequate levels of these two nutrients.

A calcium and vitamin D supplement can increase your bone density and reduce your risk of bone fracture. A gluten-free diet will help your small intestine heal so that it can absorb calcium and vitamin D from the food you eat and the beverages you drink. Gluten-free sources of calcium and vitamin D include milk and some milk substitutes, as well as fatty fish. Tofu, beans, and leafy greens such as spinach, kale and broccoli are high in calcium.

If you can't eat or drink dairy products, or if testing indicates that you're deficient in calcium, your dietitian may recommend taking a gluten-free calcium supplement (1,200 milligrams) that also contains vitamin D (600 to 800 international units) each day. In some cases, higher dosages may be appropriate. If you need to take higher doses, it's important that your doctor monitor your blood and, sometimes, urine levels to make sure you're not getting too much.

Follow-up visits

After your initial diagnosis, you'll likely come back for a follow-up visit with your doctor three to six months later. During this visit, your doctor will want to assess your symptoms and see how you're doing with your diet. Typically, you'll have some bloodwork done at this time.

Depending on your circumstances, your doctor may request a bone density scan if you haven't already had one to assess the health of your bones. Another goal of a follow-up visit is to make sure you're not experiencing any complications.

BLOOD TESTS Follow-up blood tests will measure levels of antibodies associated with celiac disease. Typically the deamidated gliadin peptide (DGP-IgA plus DGP-IgG) test or the tissue transglutaminase antibody (tTG-IgA) test is performed. The results are compared with your original baseline tests when the disease was first diagnosed.

Follow-up blood tests let your doctor know if your diet is working and if antibody levels are declining. These tests won't detect very small amounts of gluten, but they're pretty good indicators of whether harmful amounts are still getting into your system.

Your doctor may also request blood tests to check that any nutritional deficiencies are improving.

ANNUAL CHECKUPS If your symptoms are better and your bloodwork shows a good response to your diet, your doctor may want to see you again in a year. At that time, he or she may want to do another bone density scan if your earlier scan indicated you have osteoporosis or are at risk.

As long as you're feeling well, your symptoms are under control, and your antibody levels are back to normal, you may only need to see a doctor once a year after the first year has passed. If you're not feeling well or have other illnesses, you may need to see your doctor more often. Persistent symptoms require additional testing (see Chapter 7).

In adults, healing typically happens much slower than in children. It's also not as complete as previously thought. As many as half of people may still have some small intestinal damage two years after starting a gluten-free diet.

At Mayo Clinic, doctors usually perform another biopsy two years after diagnosis among adults with celiac disease to make sure that healing has occurred. Some doctors don't perform repeat biopsies unless you have continued symptoms. Intestinal damage that persists may be associated with long-term risk of complications. If damage is found, it's important that you continue to be evaluated for possible complications. Your doctor or dietitian will also help you search for hidden sources of gluten contamination that may be responsible for the lack of healing.

DIETITIAN VISITS Some people find they need to see a dietitian knowledgeable about celiac disease periodically during the first year — perhaps even more frequently than they see their doctors. This is because learning the ins and outs of eating gluten-free can be tricky when first getting started.

Visiting with a dietitian can also be helpful if your bloodwork shows that you may still be eating food that contains gluten. A dietitian can go over your eating plan with you and help you check for any hidden sources of gluten — foods that you thought were gluten-free that aren't. A dietitian can also help you identify inadvertent cross-contamination. This is when gluten-free foods accidently come in contact with foods or kitchen utensils that contain gluten.

If you're feeling overwhelmed and find that you're not able to follow a gluten-free diet like you're supposed to, a dietitian can help you find ways to overcome barriers you're confronting and get you back on track. He or she

If you're around people with celiac disease often enough, you'll probably hear the term "getting glutened," a shorthand description for those times when you accidentally or unintentionally consume gluten.

Getting glutened can lead to a number of bothersome signs and symptoms, including diarrhea, bloating, fatigue and others. After you stop eating gluten, your symptoms should eventually go away. But what do you do in the meantime?

You don't have to suffer through it. It's OK to take some simple measures, including over-the-counter medications, to ease symptoms. If you have diarrhea, for example, you might take an anti-diarrheal medicine. Or if you have a headache, a pain reliever might help. Getting plenty of rest also is beneficial. If you have severe symptoms, call your doctor. He or she might recommend a short-term round of steroids to help calm the inflammation in your intestine and ease your symptoms.

may also be able to connect you with a support group, which can be a very helpful source of information and guidance.

Accidents and hidden gluten

When you're starting out — and sometimes even when you've been gluten-free for years — accidents can and do happen. You might mistakenly eat something at a party that contains gluten, or you might find that a food that was once gluten-free now contains gluten.

Often, you know something is wrong because all of a sudden your symptoms are back. You might experience abdominal pain, diarrhea or other signs and symptoms. The symptoms may feel even worse than they did before because your body has become used to being gluten-free.

Try not to fret too much — accidents happen. Pick up where you left off and keep striving to live gluten-free. As you become more experienced, you'll make fewer mistakes. You'll also know where gluten may be lurking. Gluten can sometimes be found in places you didn't expect, such as in medications.

If you find that accidents seem to happen a lot, consider reviewing your diet and daily routine with a dietitian to make sure you understand what you

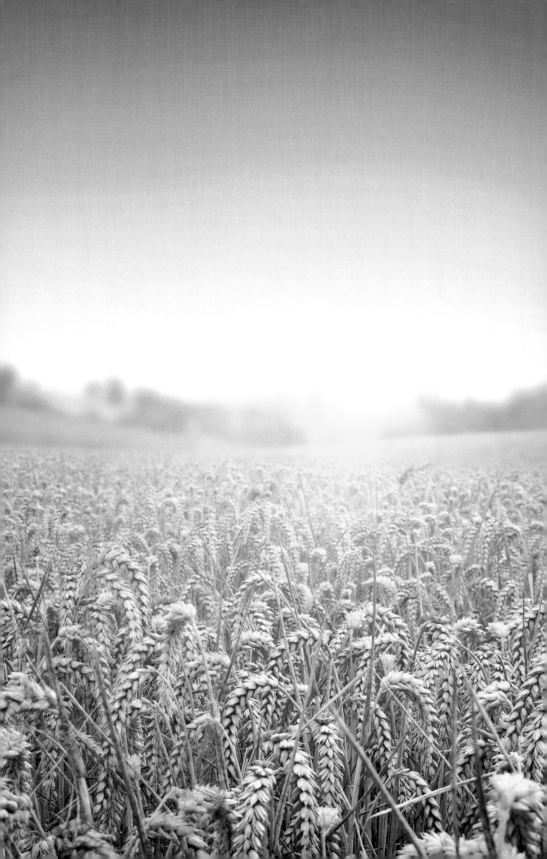

should and shouldn't eat. If symptoms develop after eating a certain food, investigate its ingredients further. It may contain gluten disguised as an ingredient you weren't familiar with or you didn't recognize.

At times, you might just feel overwhelmed by it all and give in to a momentary craving for a piece of bread or some pasta. Temptation can be difficult to handle, especially when you're hungry and if you don't have any gluten-free food handy. Of course, it's best to avoid temptation rather than to try to resist it. This may mean carrying a gluten-free snack with you almost all of the time.

If you do accidently eat a food that contains gluten, don't feel as if you need to finish it off. More is worse than less. While a bite may not be good for you, an entire helping is definitely much worse.

Depending on how your body reacts to gluten, you might feel really sick or you might feel nothing at all. Even if you feel OK, this doesn't mean it's safe to eat gluten. Even small amounts can damage your intestines, whether you feel anything or not. If you continue to eat foods that have gluten, your health problems won't improve.

On the horizon

A gluten-free diet is a safe and generally effective treatment for celiac disease. If you follow it closely, it can eliminate almost all of your symptoms and greatly reduce your risk of complications. But it's not always the easiest treatment to follow, as anyone who has to follow a gluten-free diet can tell you. In addition, for a small percentage of people, a gluten-free diet isn't enough to reverse their symptoms.

For these reasons, scientists are looking at different ways of treating celiac disease that could mean a less restrictive diet in the future. Here are some options being investigated. Currently, none have been approved for use outside of research studies.

PRETREATED GLUTEN One of the ways to avoid gluten's potentially harmful effects is to eliminate some of its damaging properties before it enters your body. Some methods to accomplish this include:
  → Development of wheat strains that don't activate the immune system
  → Adding beneficial bacteria to wheat dough to neutralize gluten proteins

The ultimate goal is to produce wheat and wheat flours with less gluten but that still retain qualities such as elasticity and tenderness. However, challenges remain with this approach, including the ability to market the product in an economy where current wheat strains are cheap and easy to grow.

DIGESTIVE ENZYMES Another approach is to take a digestive enzyme designed to help your body process gluten. One such pill developed in Europe called AN-PEP uses an enzyme from *Aspergillus niger*, a yeast that can digest gluten. Trials of this type of enzyme are in the preliminary stages.

A second example uses a combination of specifically engineered enzymes that target gluten in the intestine. It's currently being tested among volunteers with persistent symptoms despite being on a gluten-free diet.

TIGHTENING UP INTESTINAL JUNCTIONS Scientists are working on a drug (larazotide acetate) that aims to tighten up the intestinal lining so that gluten can't get through to cause problems. In people with celiac disease who are exposed to gluten, their intestinal lining goes through changes. The junctions between the cells in the lining pull apart, allowing gluten and other substances to pass through, aggravating the immune response. This is sometimes referred to as a "leaky gut."

The experimental drug works by blocking the effect of gluten, and other potentially dangerous messengers called cytokines, at the junctions between cells. This reduces the passage of gluten across the intestinal lining barrier.

BLOCKING GLUTEN'S ENTRY With this approach, scientists are looking into using a substance that binds to certain gluten molecules (peptides) within the intestine. The way the substance binds to the peptides prevents them from entering the intestinal lining and interacting with the immune system.

GLUTEN VACCINE One of the most intriguing treatments is that of a gluten vaccine. It's possible that people with celiac disease either never developed a tolerance for gluten in early life or they lost the ability to tolerate gluten later as adults.

Studies are underway to see if injection of a protein-based vaccine helps people with the gene most commonly associated with celiac disease (HLA-DQ2) rebuild their tolerance to gluten.

The idea behind the vaccine is that it would desensitize the body to gluten, similar to how allergy shots work. Initial shots contain just enough gluten to tease the immune system and fool it into ignoring the gluten — but not enough to cause a full-blown reaction. Over time, the dose of gluten may be increased or repeated frequently. If successful, the shots might allow people with celiac disease to build up a tolerance to gluten, eventually allowing them to eat a normal diet.

Only time and several studies will tell if a gluten vaccine or other types of treatments could be a passport to eating gluten without experiencing punishment to your gut.

When symptoms persist

Occasionally — estimates are between 7 and 30 percent of the time — symptoms persist even after following a gluten-free diet. If this happens to you, you and your doctor, and often a dietitian, need to take a close look at your diet. One of the most common reasons symptoms linger is because small amounts of gluten are still being ingested, and you don't know it.

Less commonly, symptoms recur or persist even when all gluten is removed from the diet. In this case, additional tests may be needed to determine if you have other health problems. Medication or other types of treatment also may be necessary.

The next chapter will help you understand what happens when symptoms don't respond to a gluten-free diet.

CHAPTER SEVEN

When treatment doesn't work

You started on a gluten-free diet, and you've followed it faithfully for six months or maybe even a year. Yet you still have diarrhea, bloating and gas. And you continue to feel tired and lethargic. Weren't all, or at least most, of these symptoms supposed to go away by now? What's up?

While most people with celiac disease respond to a gluten-free diet within a few weeks, a sizable percentage — up to 30 percent by some estimates — continue to have symptoms six to 12 months later. In some cases, the symptoms initially go away and then come back. In other cases, they never really resolve. Doctors refer to this as nonresponsive celiac disease — celiac disease that doesn't respond to a gluten-free diet. Other signs of non-responsive celiac disease include persistently elevated antibody levels and intestinal damage that doesn't heal in spite of gluten avoidance.

Everyone recovers from celiac symptoms at a different rate. And it's true that some aspects of the disease take longer than others to resolve. For example, skin rashes (dermatitis herpetiformis) may take a year or longer to clear up. Loss of bone density and tingling in your hands and feet (peripheral neuropathy) may never go away completely. However, if you've been strictly gluten-free for six months to a year and you're not really feeling better, it's important to let your doctor know.

The most common reason symptoms persist or recur is because somehow gluten is still getting into your diet. A dietitian can do a careful review of what and where you eat, medications you take, and your risk of gluten exposure at work or home, to look for hidden sources.

Occasionally, it turns out that the diagnosis is wrong. It's not celiac disease but something else causing the intestinal damage. It can also happen that another disorder has developed alongside celiac disease — such as microscopic colitis or an overgrowth of bacteria in the digestive system — that also needs to be treated.

For a very small percentage of people with celiac disease, even very careful avoidance of gluten isn't enough to heal the intestine and provide relief from symptoms. This is called refractory celiac disease (refractory sprue). For people with refractory celiac disease, additional specialized treatment is needed.

Another look

If you continue to experience symptoms of celiac disease despite being on a gluten-free diet for several months or your symptoms come back, the first step your doctor may want to take is to go back and review your initial diagnosis. He or she may want to make sure that your initial blood tests and biopsy results truly reflect celiac disease.

Is it refractory celiac disease?

A doctor will generally follow these steps before concluding that a person has refractory celiac disease.

- Reconfirm test results for celiac disease.

- Check for hidden gluten.

- Check for lactose intolerance, bacterial overgrowth of the small intestine, microscopic colitis and pancreatic insufficiency.

- Check for irritable bowel syndrome or other dietary issues, including a carbohydrate intolerance known as FODMAPs (see page 132).

- If above conditions are absent, test results are negative, and intestinal damage persists, assume it's refractory celiac disease.

If there are any uncertainties, your doctor may request an endoscopy procedure with biopsies to see if your intestine is healing. He or she may also look for clues in your medical and family history that might provide helpful insight. This might include checking to see if any of your relatives has celiac disease or if you or one of your relatives has an autoimmune disorder associated with celiac disease, such as type 1 diabetes or thyroid disease.

If your doctor feels confident that you have celiac disease, you'll likely be referred to a dietitian for a thorough dietary review. If there's doubt as to whether celiac disease is truly the culprit, the next step is to search for other causes of your symptoms.

IS GLUTEN STILL BEING INGESTED? If your doctor is fairly certain that you have celiac disease, he or she will want you to see a dietitian familiar with celiac disease and who understands the complexities of living gluten-free. Most of the time, the reason that people with celiac disease continue to experience symptoms is because they're still ingesting gluten in one form or another.

Your dietitian may ask you to complete a survey or keep a food journal for a period of time to assess your eating habits and look for other lifestyle patterns that may inadvertently be exposing you to gluten. If you eat out often or you don't always read labels, you may unknowingly be coming into contact with gluten. Perhaps the vitamin supplement you take contains gluten. Or maybe it's something else you ingest, such as the communion wafer at church.

People often think they're doing a good job avoiding all gluten, but blood tests indicate they're still ingesting gluten. Your dietitian can help you discover possible sources of gluten that you may not be aware of.

In addition, some people react to even minuscule amounts of gluten. It's difficult, if not impossible, to avoid at least some cross-contamination between foods that don't contain gluten and those that do. This may be true not only in restaurants but also in your own home. Most people with celiac disease are generally able to tolerate these very small amounts, but some people cannot. Although you're technically eating gluten-free, you may still be ingesting enough gluten to make you sick.

In one research study, individuals with nonresponsive celiac disease were prescribed a modified gluten-free diet called the Gluten Contamination Elimination Diet. This diet, in which volunteers were followed for three to six months, was designed to avoid any kind of cross-contamination. It consisted of only fresh, whole foods, such as fresh fruits and vegetables and unprocessed meats. No grains were allowed except for brown or white rice.

Before starting the diet, all of the 17 volunteers except for one had persistent celiac symptoms, including diarrhea, fatigue and abdominal pain.

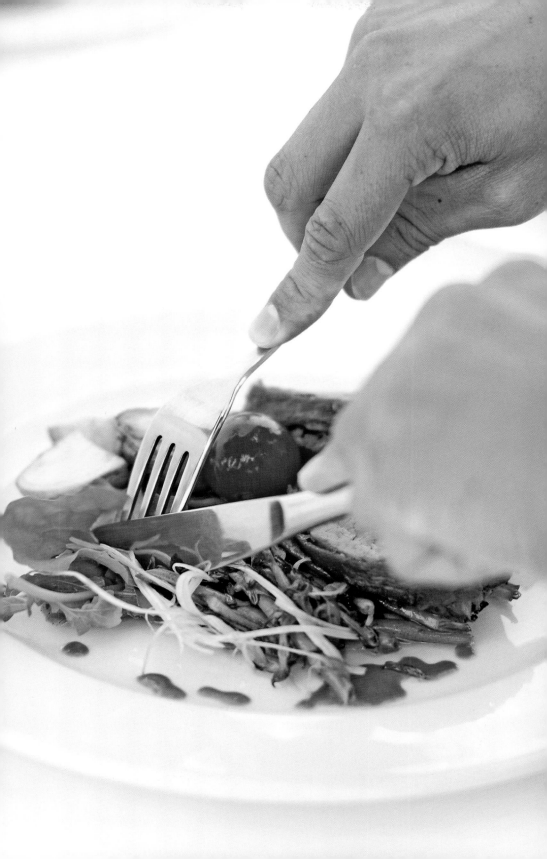

Of those who completed the diet, 14 experienced relief from their symptoms and 11 of the 14 were able to return to a regular gluten-free diet without recurrence of symptoms. Among most of the volunteers, antibody levels returned to normal and intestinal healing occurred.

What researchers learned from this study is that people with celiac disease who don't respond to a regular gluten-free diet may in fact be sensitive to even very small amounts of gluten. For these people, it's important that they follow a diet that avoids all processed foods, and stay with the diet long enough to allow the intestine to heal.

WAS THE ORIGINAL DIAGNOSIS WRONG? In some cases, the reason for continued symptoms is because the original diagnosis was incorrect. A misdiagnosis is more common when it's based on antibody test results alone without a follow-up biopsy of the small intestine. It may also be wrong if the diagnosis was made because symptoms initially improved after eliminating gluten and no actual testing was done. An intestinal biopsy is generally a reliable indicator of celiac disease, but if the original results were borderline abnormal, there's a possibility the diagnosis was made incorrectly.

If your doctor has doubts about your original diagnosis, he or she may ask you to undergo genetic testing (see page 70) or do a gluten challenge. For this test, you introduce gluten back into your diet for a period of time, followed by a repeat biopsy to evaluate the effects of gluten on your small intestine (see page 72).

If after a gluten challenge the biopsy results show signs of inflammation and damaged villi, celiac disease is typically confirmed. Your doctor will likely recommend that you go back on a gluten-free diet under the supervision of an experienced dietitian. If the biopsy shows no intestinal damage, then gluten probably isn't the cause of your symptoms. The next step is to look for another cause.

IS A DIFFERENT DISEASE RESPONSIBLE? If biopsy results show that you have intestinal inflammation and damaged villi and a careful dietary review has eliminated any known trace of gluten, it's possible you may have a condition that's not celiac disease. Other diseases can also damage and inflame your intestinal lining, although they're not nearly as common as celiac disease.

One such disease is tropical sprue, an illness characterized by chronic diarrhea, intestinal damage and malabsorption. It's mainly acquired in certain tropical areas, specifically Central and South America and Southeast Asia.

Crohn's disease, an inflammatory bowel disorder, generally affects the lower small intestine or the colon or both. Rarely, it can develop in the upper and middle small intestine and produce symptoms similar to celiac disease. Although uncommon, some people can have both Crohn's disease and celiac disease.

Other possible conditions include a parasite infection (giardiasis); a disease that causes thickening of the intestine lining called collagenous sprue; a bacterial infection called Whipple's disease; and an autoimmune disorder that usually occurs in infants but can also develop in adults (autoimmune enteropathy). Some medications also can damage the small intestine, and certain immune deficiencies may produce symptoms that mimic celiac disease.

IS THERE AN ADDITIONAL PROBLEM? Sometimes symptoms persist because another gastrointestinal disorder may develop alongside celiac disease. It's the other disorder, not celiac disease, that's responsible for the ongoing symptoms. Some conditions that may occur along with celiac disease include:

Lactose or fructose intolerance Lactose or fructose intolerance may occur as a result of, or along with, celiac disease. Lactose intolerance is a condition that develops when your small intestine cannot tolerate the natural sugar (lactose) in milk and other dairy products. Fructose intolerance results when your small intestine can't properly absorb fructose, a sugar found naturally in fruits and honey. Fructose is also found in processed foods such as table sugar and high-fructose corn syrup.

Because lactose intolerance is common in people with celiac disease, your doctor or dietitian may recommend that you avoid dairy products when first starting a gluten-free diet. Once your small intestine has had time to heal and normal absorptive functions have returned, then you can start eating dairy products again.

If your symptoms return when you resume eating foods containing lactose or fructose, talk to your doctor or a dietitian. You may need to avoid lactose or fructose for a longer period or limit them indefinitely.

Irritable bowel syndrome Irritable bowel syndrome (IBS) is a common disorder that affects the intestines. It causes signs and symptoms similar to celiac disease, such as cramping, abdominal pain, bloating, gas, diarrhea and constipation. It's not uncommon for the two to be mistaken for each other. However, they can also occur together. Your doctor may determine that your continued symptoms are related to IBS, not celiac disease.

Your doctor can help you learn how to manage IBS. Most people with IBS find that their symptoms improve as they learn to manage their diets and lifestyles and find healthy ways to deal with stress.

Rapid transit With this condition, food is dumped out of the stomach too quickly and it passes through the small intestine too rapidly. Because of the rapid transit, the small intestine isn't able to digest the food and absorb nutrients and water as it normally should. This can lead to incomplete digestion and diarrhea, but usually doesn't cause nutrient malabsorption.

Bacterial overgrowth A variety of healthy bacteria live in your digestive tract. Most are in your colon with a smaller percentage in your small intestine. Your body keeps the number of bacteria in check, but sometimes an overgrowth of bacteria can occur in the small intestine. This overgrowth can produce inflammation and trigger signs and symptoms such as bloating, gas, abdominal discomfort and, occasionally, watery diarrhea.

It's not uncommon for people with celiac disease to develop bacterial overgrowth in the small intestine. However, because both conditions have similar symptoms, it can be difficult to distinguish between the two. To treat bacterial overgrowth and return bacteria to a normal level, antibiotics are prescribed.

Microscopic colitis If one of your main problems is chronic diarrhea, your doctor may request a biopsy of your colon to check for microscopic colitis. Microscopic colitis is a subtle inflammation of your colon that can only be seen through a microscope. It's not clear what causes microscopic colitis, but people with celiac disease have a much higher risk of developing it than do people who don't have celiac disease.

Anti-diarrheal medications, such as Imodium and Pepto-Bismol, can help treat microscopic colitis. Steroids that work on the lining of the colon can help reduce and control the inflammation. Sometimes stopping a medication that may be unrelated to celiac disease can help.

Pancreatic insufficiency Some people with celiac disease experience inflammation of the pancreas. This happens because the damaged small intestine isn't able to signal the pancreas that food is on its way, so that the pancreas can produce and release digestive juices (enzymes) needed for digestion. As a result, food isn't broken down and digested properly. This is known as pancreatic insufficiency.

Signs and symptoms associated with pancreatic insufficiency include diarrhea, gas and bloating. If your doctor suspects you may have a problem with your pancreas, he or she may request tests to check that it's functioning properly. Pancreatic insufficiency is usually treated with prescription enzyme supplements to make up for the deficiency. Over-the-counter digestive enzymes aren't helpful.

Refractory celiac disease

A few people with celiac disease — about 1 to 2 percent of those who are diagnosed — continue to experience symptoms despite eliminating all gluten from their diets. Biopsies of the small intestine continue to show severe damage a year after the disease was diagnosed, and symptoms may be just as bad or even worse. Further examination and additional tests aren't able to uncover any other cause for the continued symptoms. These people are considered to have refractory celiac disease (refractory sprue).

Refractory celiac disease (RCD) is rare and generally occurs in adults older than age 50. Signs and symptoms are typically more severe than those associated with uncomplicated celiac disease. They often include severe weight loss, malnutrition, and multiple vitamin and mineral deficiencies.

Why RCD develops is unclear. It may have to do with an increased genetic predisposition toward the disease. People with two copies of the genetic variants needed to develop celiac disease seem to be more likely to have RCD than are those with only one copy. This is true at least in some European countries. RCD also may result from living with the disease and eating gluten for many years before the disease is finally diagnosed. More research is needed to understand what prompts RCD to occur.

There are two types of refractory celiac disease:

* **Type 1.** Type 1 is much like uncomplicated celiac disease, except that it doesn't respond to eliminating gluten from your diet. With type 1, key immune cells in the intestinal lining (lymphocytes) retain their normal appearance.

* **Type 2.** With type 2 disease, changes occur to the lymphocytes. They display abnormalities that may be precancerous, increasing your risk of intestinal cancer. These abnormal cells can be detected through laboratory analysis of a biopsy sample.

TREATMENT Although there's no treatment that can cure RCD, it's still recommended that you avoid all gluten to prevent potentially greater complications.

Additional goals of treatment are to provide nutritional support and reduce inflammation of the intestinal lining. Nutritional supplements can help correct nutritional deficiencies; however, sometimes it's necessary to receive nutrients intravenously. This may first happen at a hospital and later at home.

Steroid medications may be prescribed to help control inflammation of the intestinal lining. In most people with type 1 RCD, steroids can relieve symptoms and they may even allow the intestine to heal. With type 2 disease, steroids may improve symptoms but they usually don't lead to complete recovery from intestinal damage. Type 2 disease can progress to cancer of the small intestine, so ongoing care and surveillance are needed.

If steroids aren't helpful, medications to suppress an overactive immune system may ease symptoms and reduce inflammation for people with type 1 RCD. However, these medications can produce severe side effects, such as a weakened immune system and an increased risk of infection. Immunosuppressive therapy generally isn't recommended for people with type 2 RCD because it can accelerate the progression of cancer of the intestinal lining.

In the meantime, new treatments are being developed to help people with persistent or recurring symptoms. These treatments are intended to be used in conjunction with a gluten-free diet.

COMPLICATIONS Refractory celiac disease can lead to a number of complications. Malnutrition is common, and it can be fatal. In addition, individuals with RCD are very prone to infections. Among people with type 2 RCD, large sores can develop along the intestinal lining (ulcerative jejunitis), along with other intestinal abnormalities, including blockages (strictures).

Treatment may involve surgery to remove the damaged section of the small intestine. If the damage is limited to one part of the intestine, removal of the damaged section may lead to long-term improvement, although it's still important to follow a gluten-free diet.

Cancer Celiac disease is also associated with increased risk of several types of cancer. Most common is cancer of the intestinal lining (intestinal lymphoma). Most people with type 1 RCD don't develop lymphoma, although a few do. However, about one-third to one-half of people with type 2 RCD develop lymphoma within the first five years of diagnosis. This is probably because of the precancerous changes that have already occurred in some of their immune cells. That's why regular monitoring for the development of lymphoma is critical. Among some individuals, only after they're diagnosed with cancer do they learn they have celiac disease.

Treatment may involve surgery or chemotherapy drugs, but they're not always effective. Generally the more widespread the cancer is when it's first discovered, the more difficult it is to treat. In addition, some individuals are too ill to withstand the treatment. Scientists continue to explore other potential treatment options, including combination of chemotherapy and stem cell transplantation.

COPING Coping with persistent symptoms can be exhausting — mentally, emotionally and physically. You've probably seen multiple doctors and dietitians and had more tests than you care to remember. Dealing with a chronic illness isn't easy, especially when things get complicated. In addition to seeing your doctor for regular checkups, you may find it helpful to lean on others for support.

One way to do this is through a support group for people with celiac disease. Ask your doctor or dietitian for a recommendation or visit some of the associations listed at the end of this book that offer online support groups (see pages 274 and 275). Try to stay positive and take things one step at a time.

Related Conditions

CHAPTER EIGHT

A spectrum of disorders

Let's begin with some of what we know about gluten and wheat. Scientists know that consuming gluten — a protein found in wheat, barley and rye — can cause celiac disease in some people. Celiac disease results from an autoimmune response, a condition in which your own immune system is harming you. In the case of celiac disease, when you eat foods that contain gluten, your immune system responds to the gluten the same as it does a foreign invader — it tries to attack and destroy it. The trouble is, your small intestine pays the price. The disease damages the lining of the small intestine and prevents it from properly digesting and absorbing nutrients in food.

Scientists also know that some people experience an allergic response when they eat food made from wheat, what's known as wheat allergy. Wheat allergy is sometimes confused with celiac disease, but the two conditions are actually very different. Unlike celiac disease, which produces a variety of signs and symptoms, including abdominal pain and diarrhea, signs and symptoms of wheat allergy are similar to other allergic responses. They generally include hives and skin rash, swelling of the lips and tongue, sneezing, watery eyes, difficulty breathing, and less often, gastrointestinal symptoms.

Wheat allergy occurs when any part of the wheat kernel is consumed, and the response is immediate — symptoms often develop within seconds to minutes. Celiac disease, on the other hand, is specific to one component of

Gluten- and wheat-related disorders

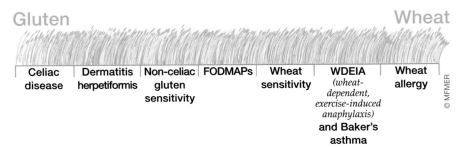

Gluten   Wheat

Celiac disease	Dermatitis herpetiformis	Non-celiac gluten sensitivity	FODMAPs	Wheat sensitivity	WDEIA *(wheat-dependent, exercise-induced anaphylaxis)* and Baker's asthma	Wheat allergy

© MFMER

When you picture all of the gluten- and wheat-related conditions lined up in a row, you'll find celiac disease on one end and wheat allergy on the other. In the middle are a number of other conditions that researchers are trying to learn more about.

wheat — gluten — which is also found in barley and rye (see "What's in a wheat kernel?" on page 118). With celiac disease, it often takes hours or days after gluten is consumed for a response to occur.

Celiac disease and wheat allergy represent the ends of a spectrum. Both conditions have been studied extensively for many years. Researchers know what causes them, what may increase your risk of getting them, and how to diagnose and treat them. In the case of celiac disease, you can't eat anything that contains gluten, and in the case of wheat allergy, you can't eat anything made from wheat.

In the middle of the spectrum are some emerging conditions — commonly referred to as sensitivities — that are gathering an increasing amount of attention. These conditions make up a murky middle ground. They represent individuals who don't have celiac disease or who aren't allergic to wheat, but who are bothered after eating foods containing gluten or made from wheat.

There's a lot about these disorders that researchers don't know. However, scientists are working to try to find some answers. In this section of the book, we'll talk about gluten and wheat sensitivities and the growing movement to avoid gluten even among people who are healthy.

The spectrum widens

A lot has changed in just a couple of decades. Once thought to be a relatively rare disease outside of Europe, celiac disease can now be found worldwide. And the number of people being diagnosed with the disease is increasing every year.

Wheat kernels have several different parts, all of which may play a different role in gluten- or wheat-related disorders. The entire wheat kernel is the seed from which wheat grows. When sold as food, entire kernels are often called wheat berries. Inside each kernel, there are three components.

Germ. A tiny portion of the total weight of the kernel (2.5 percent), the germ is the sprouting portion of the seed. Because it contains about 10 percent fat, which would interfere with baking, it's usually separated from the rest of the kernel when milling wheat into flour.

Endosperm. This portion of the kernel contains most of its weight (83 percent) and is made up of protein (gluten), carbohydrates, iron, digestible (soluble) fiber and B vitamins. The endosperm is the main component of flour, and contains the most gluten of any component of the wheat kernel.

Bran. This component of the kernel includes its outer shell. It makes up 14 percent of the kernel's weight, and is included in whole-wheat flour, but not white flour. It contains indigestible (insoluble) fiber that has laxative properties. Many nutrients and other beneficial substances associated with eating whole-wheat foods are derived from the bran.

Wheat kernel

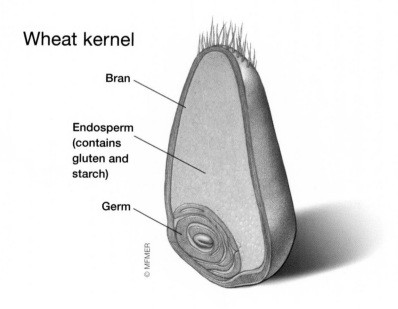

Bran

Endosperm
(contains
gluten and
starch)

Germ

© MFMER

At the same time, scientists are learning that gluten or another component of wheat may be responsible for other conditions that are different from celiac disease or wheat allergy but that often produce some of the same symptoms.

The foundation for these emerging disorders took place in the 1980s. Studies were published about individuals who didn't have celiac disease — they tested negative for the disease — but who still exhibited celiac-like symptoms. And similar to celiac disease, their symptoms improved on a gluten-free diet. The studies provided little in the way of solid answers other than the fact that participants felt better after they had eliminated gluten from their diets.

Many questions began to emerge. If the study participants' symptoms couldn't be explained as an autoimmune response (celiac disease) or as an allergic response (wheat allergy), what could be causing them? The idea that some people may have "a sensitivity" to gluten took hold. Interestingly, the more researchers began to explore the concept of gluten sensitivity, the more it became clear that gluten might not always be the culprit. In other words, it quickly became evident there wasn't a one-size-fits-all answer to these people's troubles.

Here's an example. You've been tested for celiac disease, and test results show that you don't have it. But after eating certain foods, such as bread or pasta, you typically experience belly pain, gas or loose stools. When you don't eat those foods, you feel better. So what's going on? There is a range of possibilities:

❈ You may be sensitive to gluten, a condition commonly known as non-celiac gluten sensitivity.

❈ You may be sensitive to other components of wheat, not specifically gluten, what's often referred to as wheat sensitivity.

❈ You may be sensitive to other substances in the foods you eat, specifically a group of carbohydrates that don't digest well in the small intestine. FODMAPs is the name for these carbohydrates, one of which (fructan) is found in wheat, barley and rye.

❈ You may have another disorder such as inflammatory bowel disease in which certain foods, including those that contain wheat, may play a role in your symptoms.

In the chapters that follow, you'll learn more about the conditions and disorders that make up the gluten- and wheat-related spectrum. Keep in mind that some of these conditions aren't clearly defined. Here are some general descriptions to help you navigate the murky waters.

Non-celiac gluten sensitivity. This term is generally used to describe individuals who don't test positive for celiac disease, but who have symptoms that seem to coincide with celiac disease. Some doctors use the term *celiac-lite* to describe this condition. People with non-celiac gluten sensitivity experience symptoms that coincide with eating gluten, similar to people with celiac disease. But unlike celiac disease, blood tests don't reveal specific antibodies associated with the disease (see page 63) and standard tests don't find any intestinal damage. These individuals may or may not have the genetic makeup for celiac disease.

Wheat sensitivity. Wheat sensitivity is a term used to describe individuals who experience specific symptoms after eating products made from wheat. They don't have celiac disease, and they differ from individuals with non-celiac gluten sensitivity in that their symptoms tend to be more diverse, including headaches, joint pain and "foggy" brain. Their symptoms also seem to be more closely tied to eating wheat rather than products made from barley and

Sifting through the confusion

Researchers continue to study and learn more about the wheat- and gluten-related conditions on the spectrum. It's a complicated task, not only because the conditions share so many features but also because of the immense variation of symptoms. It's difficult to label any single case as typical or conventional.

In addition, with the exception of celiac disease and wheat allergy, there are few tests that can confirm gluten or wheat sensitivity or FODMAPs. The conditions are generally diagnosed through a process of exclusion — if it looks like you don't have condition X and you don't have condition Y, then the explanation of your symptoms may lie with condition Z. This intuitive process has created doubts among some scientists about whether some of the conditions even exist. (Two food sensitivities for which tests are available are lactose and fructose, two of the FODMAP carbohydrates.)

rye. The condition may not be related to eating gluten but rather other components of wheat.

FODMAPs. This acronym describes a small group of carbohydrates and related substances found in a variety of foods, including wheat, rye and barley, that can cause excessive gas, bloating, cramps and diarrhea — symptoms similar to gluten and wheat sensitivity. FODMAPs are discussed in more detail on page 132.

Wheat allergy. Wheat allergy causes an inflammatory reaction that occurs after eating foods made from wheat. Signs and symptoms generally include rash, hives, sneezing, coughing and asthma. In extreme cases, the allergy can produce life-threatening swelling of your airways (anaphylaxis).

WDEIA. This acronym stands for wheat-dependent, exercise-induced anaphylaxis, a rare form of wheat allergy that can occur during exercise shortly after eating wheat.

Baker's asthma. This is another rare form of wheat allergy that occurs when you inhale, not eat, the proteins found in flour made from wheat, rye and barley.

Another obstacle to understanding these disorders is a lack of consistent terminology. Different individuals in different locations use different terms to describe the same condition, in some cases with only slight variation and in other cases with completely different wording.

This lack of definition prompted the commission of an international task force to address the problem. The participants, all of whom were experts on wheat- and gluten-related conditions, conducted a broad survey of scientific literature, and analyzed the terminology appearing in these publications. They then recommended precise definitions and usage of various terms. Their conclusions, published in 2013 after a meeting in Oslo, Norway, are referred to as the Oslo recommendations.

This book tries to follow the Oslo recommendations, but keep in mind there's still much more to learn about wheat- and gluten-related conditions and changes in terminology are likely in the coming years.

Going against the grain

Is it a coincidence that as wheat production and consumption have increased worldwide so has the incidence of gluten- and wheat-related disorders, including the number of people diagnosed with celiac disease? Likely not.

In the last few decades, food scientists have found ways to dramatically increase the yield of wheat plants. Because of this, more wheat is available worldwide. In parts of the world in which wheat hasn't historically been a key part of the daily diet, such as China or Mexico, wheat consumption has skyrocketed. In India and some African and Latin American countries, the cultivation of wheat has caused a significant increase in the amount of food available — sometimes saving entire populations from starvation.

In addition to the increased availability of wheat, there's debate whether changes to the wheat kernel — changes in how the plant is bred — have affected its digestibility. Some researchers believe the composition of the wheat plant has changed very little over the centuries, but not all agree.

There are many theories being proposed with not a lot of science to back them up. One is that changes to the endosperm of the wheat kernel have boosted the gluten content of wheat. Another theory is that today's wheat produces softer flours, altering its gluten content. There's also the fact that many of today's foods contain more additives, including carbohydrates and gluten, that make them softer in texture and help them to rise better. These are qualities that food processors, retailers and consumers want.

What has resulted is a tension between the health benefits and the health risks of added gluten in the diet, a struggle that's been compounded by the food industry. With so many products these days touting the fact that they're gluten-free, a common assumption among the general public is that gluten must be bad for you. As a result, many people who are healthy are going out of their way to keep gluten off their plates. They wrongly assume that if people with celiac disease need to eliminate gluten to protect their health, then they should do the same thing.

A closer look

Celiac disease is discussed in Part 1 of this book. The remaining chapters in Part 2 are devoted to the other conditions on the spectrum. In the chapters that follow, you'll learn more about non-celiac gluten sensitivity, FODMAPs, wheat sensitivity, wheat allergy and unique forms of wheat allergy.

As you read the chapters, try to keep an open mind. It's easy to point to one food or a food group as the source of your symptoms. But what researchers are learning is the world of wheat and gluten is complex. It often takes time and patience, and help from a doctor or dietitian, to find the right answers.

RICK'S STORY

For well over 10 years, I had constant reflux issues and needed an antacid every night. I had a bowel movement after every single meal, and I would experience intense heartburn with certain combinations of foods. On occasion, I would throw up, but more often I just felt sick.

I'm a medical researcher by profession, and I spent years altering the food in my diet to try to figure out what was causing my symptoms. About a year ago, I read a book that linked symptoms like mine to eating wheat. To be honest, I thought the idea was rubbish, but I decided it would be an interesting experiment to cut out all food containing wheat for a week or two to see what would happen. I was also looking for a reason to eat healthier so I could lose some weight. Despite being an active person, I was overweight. So, I gave it a try.

I soon had no more diarrhea and no more upset stomach. I no longer needed an antacid each night, and I lost weight. What started as a one-week experiment grew into a monthlong transformation. We took a road trip during this first month, and I came to appreciate how much of our food was served in a bun!

I decided to contact a doctor to discuss my findings, and he suggested that I be tested for celiac disease. My tests all came back negative, but my doctor recommended that I not only continue to eliminate wheat but that I avoid all foods containing gluten, if I could make it work. This was a total paradigm shift in my mind. My whole life, I thought you were supposed to eat according to the food pyramid, which is basically stacked on top of wheat.

I've been on a gluten-free diet for a year now, and I find it to be very satisfying. I've continued to lose weight, be healthy and be symptom-free. It's hard to know if the difference is completely due to avoiding gluten or just avoiding processed foods and consuming fewer calories, but I enjoy the change.

I do experience symptoms when I make a mistake or I consume trace amounts of gluten. So I'm very careful about what I eat. I remain an avid label reader, and I'm fortunate that I actually enjoy cooking. Breakfast is usually simple. I eat scrambled eggs practically every day with a side of fruit or salsa and a small side of meat. Lunch and dinner are usually "meat and threes" — some kind of meat with two or three vegetables or a side salad. I'm from the South and "meat and threes" is a way of life in the South, so it works well for me. For lunch, I choose meat and three from the cafeteria at work. For dinner, I make meat and threes myself. We also enjoy eating out.

It's fair to say I'm relieved that I don't have celiac disease. I find it rewarding that I'm making this choice myself, rather than eating this way because I have to. I've changed my ideas about healthy eating and reconnected with real food. If you walk into a farmers market with an appetite and look at the things around you, that's what I'm eating now.

CHAPTER NINE

Non-celiac gluten sensitivity

Adam is certain something isn't right, and he thinks it's related to his diet. Not long after he eats, his gut hurts, he feels bloated, and he often has gas. These symptoms don't happen every time he eats but often enough. Several visits with his doctor haven't come up with a cause. He's been tested for celiac disease, but tests showed he doesn't have it.

Adam has noticed a curious pattern. Saturday and Sunday are typically his days to relax. He tends to stick around the house and eat something light, often nothing more than a salad or something off the grill. On Monday mornings, he feels pretty good — the best he'll feel all week. At work he often has lunch at a nearby restaurant or fast-food place up the street. Soon after, his symptoms tend to return. And they often worsen if he joins his friends for a beer after work. The pain, bloating and gas often stay with him for the rest of the week.

Adam knows he doesn't have celiac disease because he's been tested, but he read about a condition called gluten sensitivity, and it just seemed like the article was telling his story. After all, what he typically orders for lunch is a sandwich, and there's gluten in beer, too. After visiting his doctor, Adam decided to test the idea by eliminating foods from his diet that contained gluten. Doing so has been challenging, but he's started to notice improvements in how he feels. Adam believes he may be sensitive to gluten, a condition better known in the medical community as non-celiac gluten sensitivity.

Beyond celiac disease

As you learned in the first part of this book, celiac disease is an autoimmune disorder. It results when your immune system responds to gluten in the food you eat the same as it does a foreign invader — it tries to attack and destroy it. This constant attack every time you eat irritates and inflames your small intestine, causing gastrointestinal problems and a variety of other symptoms. Celiac disease is fairly well-understood. Doctors know the genetic makeup that puts people at risk and the mechanisms that trigger it — mainly eating food that has gluten in it. There are also specific tests that can identify if you have it.

A lot of attention has been given to celiac disease recently because it's an illness on the rise — its prevalence is increasing worldwide. However, as researchers have been learning more about gluten and the negative impact it has on the health of some individuals, the existence of another condition has gradually come into focus. Non-celiac gluten sensitivity (NCGS) describes a disorder related to, but separate from, celiac disease. NCGS may be even more common than celiac disease, but unlike celiac disease, doctors know little about it.

In fact, there's considerable debate in medical circles if NCGS even exists. Could the symptoms that people attribute to gluten and NCGS stem from another disease or disorder? Is gluten the true culprit, or might it be some other component of wheat? Is it possible it's neither gluten nor wheat but another substance commonly found in foods containing gluten? Or could it be another medical condition affecting the gut, such as irritable bowel syndrome?

What's interesting is that NCGS — often simply referred to as gluten sensitivity — is a major factor behind the current gluten-free craze. It's why you're seeing gluten-free sections in grocery stores, gluten-free meals on restaurant menus, and gluten-free logos and claims on everything from fresh meat to crackers and cookies. As the food industry realized that gluten was being targeted for an increasing number of health problems, it quickly took steps to provide gluten-free alternatives.

In the pages that follow, you'll learn about how NCGS differs from celiac disease, what's known about the condition, and many questions about it that remain unanswered.

What is NCGS?

Non-celiac gluten sensitivity is the term used to describe individuals who experience symptoms similar to celiac disease when they eat foods containing gluten. But unlike celiac disease, blood tests don't reveal the presence of specific antibodies associated with celiac disease and examination of the small intestine doesn't reveal any inflammation and damage. NCGS and celiac disease share many of the same symptoms, but NCGS is believed to be less severe than celiac disease. Sometimes the disease is referred to as "celiac-lite."

There is no test for NCGS. When someone is diagnosed with the condition, it's generally after tests for other conditions that may produce similar symptoms — including celiac disease — come back negative. An elimination diet may also be recommended before a diagnosis is made. With this test, you eliminate all gluten from your diet for a short period of time to see if your symptoms improve, and then reintroduce gluten back into your diet to see if they worsen (see page 130). If you aren't eating gluten, your symptoms should disappear. If they don't go away, then the problem isn't gluten.

Treatment of NCGS is similar to that of celiac disease. Both involve eliminating gluten from your diet. The difference is with celiac disease it's essential to avoid all traces of gluten — because gluten is what's destroying the lining of your small intestine and opening up the possibility of other serious complications. With NCGS, there's no damage occurring to your small intestine, so you may be able to eat some gluten. Some people find they can tolerate small amounts of gluten without experiencing symptoms. How much gluten you may be able to eat depends on the type of symptoms you experience and their severity. Tolerance varies from one person to another.

WHAT'S KNOWN ABOUT NCGS Researchers have been studying non-celiac gluten sensitivity for decades, but only recently did they agree on a set of factors that must be present for an individual to be designated as having NCGS. They include the following:
  - Negative results on blood tests and an endoscopic biopsy to look for damage to the small intestine
  - An improvement in symptoms when gluten is removed from the diet, and a recurrence of symptoms when gluten is re-introduced
  - No alternative explanation for the symptoms

Celiac disease results from an autoimmune response. Your ever-vigilant immune system recognizes gluten as a foreign invader that must be destroyed instead of a food that should be digested and tolerated. It fights the gluten similar to how it responds to viruses or bacteria that need to be eliminated from your body. With NCGS, it's not clear if the symptoms people experience result from a similar type of immune response, from some type of chemical effect, or from some yet unexplained effect of gluten on digestion.

NCGS also isn't the same as wheat allergy. Wheat allergy is an allergic response that occurs when a specific substance (allergen) enters or comes into contact with your body and causes an exaggerated, immediate reaction. Common food allergens include shellfish, peanuts, milk, eggs and soy. Wheat allergy, which is discussed in the next chapter, is less common. Signs and symptoms include swelling, itching, skin rash, mouth tingling or burning, and nasal congestion. They are different than those that occur with NCGS.

The numbers on NCGS

It's not known how many people may have NCGS. Estimates vary widely, with some researchers believing it may be more common than celiac disease and others claiming it to be less. Celiac disease is estimated to affect 1.8 million people in the United States.

Most everyone will agree, however, that NCGS has garnered considerable attention, especially considering so little is known about it. Why is that? One possibility has to do with the craze over gluten and the surge in gluten-free products. Gluten is increasingly, and often incorrectly, viewed as "bad." Because of this, people who frequently experience certain symptoms after eating — from gastrointestinal problems to migraines to fatigue — are quick to question if gluten might be the cause. In addition, as researchers explore whether wheat could possibly contribute to conditions beyond celiac disease — ranging from autism to Alzheimer's disease — the attention given to gluten increases.

Factors complicating the numbers for NCGS are its wide range of symptoms and its lack of definition. Sensitivity to gluten varies greatly from person to person, triggering symptoms that range from mild to severe. Questions also remain about the precise point at which a person can be diagnosed with NCGS. The circumstances are different from celiac disease, where testing can confirm either you have the condition or you don't.

Signs and symptoms

The signs and symptoms of NCGS often mimic those of celiac disease and of irritable bowel syndrome, a condition in which your digestive system is chronically irritated due to diet, lifestyle factors or both. In fact, research has found that some people with irritable bowel syndrome experience an improvement in symptoms when they follow a gluten-free diet. This has researchers questioning if some cases of irritable bowel syndrome may be associated with NCGS.

The signs and symptoms of NCGS may be digestive in nature and include:
- Abdominal bloating, pain or discomfort
- Diarrhea

* Mucus in the stool
* Gas

Signs and symptoms may also be nondigestive in nature and include:
* Headache
* "Foggy" brain, or difficulty remembering
* Fatigue
* Joint pain
* Numbness in the legs, arms or fingers
* Balance and muscle control problems

Diagnosing NCGS

The first step in diagnosing non-celiac gluten sensitivity is to rule out other conditions that produce similar symptoms. Because the signs and symptoms of NCGS, celiac disease and irritable bowel syndrome are so similar, often the best way to start is by being tested for celiac disease. Tests are available that can determine if you have celiac disease. In the cases of NCGS and irritable bowel syndrome, there are no such tests.

Regardless of the results — whether you end up learning that you have celiac disease, irritable bowel syndrome, NCGS or another condition — getting a diagnosis is a tremendous benefit. Once your doctor knows the source of your symptoms, the two of you can work together to craft an individualized treatment plan.

A simple blood test will often indicate if you might have celiac disease. A positive result doesn't mean you have celiac disease, but it does mean that you need to have an endoscopic examination of your small intestine. During this procedure, a doctor examines the small intestine and removes small pieces of tissue (biopsies) to be examined in a laboratory. If the biopsies don't show intestinal damage, then celiac disease can be eliminated as a cause of your symptoms. The key is you have to be eating gluten for the results of these tests to be accurate. If you're not eating gluten, a doctor can't determine if you have celiac disease.

Your doctor may also check for other possible conditions that could be causing your symptoms. If tests for other conditions also come back negative, then NCGS is more likely. Some alternative medicine practitioners claim they can test for NCGS with blood, saliva or stool tests. Be aware that such tests are not scientifically valid. They've not been properly tested to see if they work.

If your doctor suspects that you may have NCGS, he or she may recommend that you try what's known as an elimination diet. In this test, you avoid anything that contains gluten for a short period of time to see if your health improves. An elimination diet is considered an essential step for determining whether you may be sensitive to gluten.

An elimination diet, however, isn't quite as simple as merely removing food that contains gluten from your meals. It's also important to determine if there may be other problem foods that might be causing your symptoms. A dietitian will want to know what you generally eat to determine if other foods may also need to be removed from your diet.

What's sometimes referred to as the nocebo effect

One reason to talk to your doctor and try to diagnose your condition before you eliminate gluten from your diet is a phenomenon known as the nocebo effect. With the nocebo effect, you have yourself convinced that a harmless substance or activity is making you ill.

In the case of gluten, you believe gluten is what's triggering your symptoms, when it really is not. Therefore, when you stop eating gluten, you think that you feel better, even though there may be no change in your condition.

What often happens is that your "relief" tends to be short-lived. Symptoms typically recur, often as strong as ever. Your attention may still remain focused on gluten rather than on other possible causes.

The nocebo effect can disguise the real cause of your symptoms and interfere with getting an accurate diagnosis.

Looking for triggers

There are various ways to approach NCGS. The way you manage the condition will depend on your signs and symptoms and their severity, your willingness to eliminate certain foods from your diet, your doctor's or dietitian's recommendations, and your personal preferences.

You may be asked to keep a food journal to monitor what you eat and make note of any signs and symptoms. This may help to reveal if gluten is causing your problems, or if other foods or beverages might be responsible. If you take part in an elimination diet, continue to record what you eat in your food journal while you're on the diet. Sometimes it's also helpful to note what you were doing and how you felt while you were eating because activities and emotions also influence digestion. Be honest in your journal, and don't disguise what you're eating or how much. A journal is only valuable if it reflects your usual behaviors.

AN ELIMINATION DIET It's possible your doctor may recommend eliminating multiple foods at the same time. Often, though, it's best when starting out just to eliminate gluten. Make sure you understand what foods do and do not contain gluten so that you know what you can and cannot eat. (See Chapter 12 for more on the basics of a gluten-free diet.) It's also important that you know what to look for on food labels to know if a food contains gluten. (See Chapter 13 for more information on reading gluten-free food labels.) You may want to stock up on gluten-free foods before starting your elimination diet to make your transition as smooth as possible.

Once you have your elimination diet plan in place, eat gluten-free for one to two months, if possible. If you think this period of time is too long, follow the diet strictly for at least two to three weeks, or as advised by your doctor. If you do eat gluten or another food you weren't supposed to — either accidentally or intentionally — be sure to make note of it in your food journal.

If your symptoms are related to gluten, you should begin to feel better soon after beginning the diet. If your symptoms persist, gluten may not be the culprit. If your symptoms worsen, contact your doctor.

COMMON ISSUES WITH ELIMINATION DIETS Although an elimination diet may be helpful in determining the cause of your symptoms, some people find following such a diet difficult. The most common issues people have are not being able to eat their favorite foods and the daily hassles of knowing what and where to eat.

Food cravings It's natural to feel somewhat deprived while you're on an elimination diet, especially if some of your favorite foods are now on your don't-eat list. You may also find that gluten-free alternatives just don't taste the same.

Social issues Expect family and friends to have many questions about why you can't eat certain foods. You'll likely find that eating out is more difficult. Preparing food at home also may be more complicated, especially if you need to prepare multiple meals to accommodate family members who still want to eat gluten.

THE RE-CHALLENGE After excluding gluten for a period of time — often a month or two — your doctor will want to try a re-challenge diet. This requires that you reintroduce foods into your diet that contain gluten. Re-challenge diets can cause discomfort because your symptoms are back. But the return of your symptoms helps confirm that gluten is the true cause of your problems.

When you undertake a re-challenge diet, the food you eat should be as pure a source of wheat as possible. For example, you might eat a matzo cracker, a wheat cracker or a piece of whole-wheat bread. This is better than a slice of pizza that has gluten in the crust but contains other ingredients that could irritate your digestive system. Do this for a day or two and see how it goes. Gradually eat more crackers or bread or add more foods that contain gluten. If your doctor has recommended eliminating more than one food, follow his or her instructions carefully when re-introducing the foods into your diet.

A re-challenge test can also help determine if you can tolerate some gluten in your diet and, if so, how much. People who have NCGS often can deal with small amounts of gluten, but they may need to limit the overall amount. Trial and error may be the best way to determine how much gluten you can tolerate without it causing symptoms. Keep in mind that the gluten you're eating is not actually harming you. Gluten causes intestinal damage in people with celiac disease but not with NCGS.

Also keep in mind that elimination diets and re-challenge diets can be affected by a variety of external factors other than what you eat. A stressful day, a new medication, poor sleep and inactivity also can affect your digestive health. You need to be patient with the process.

FUTURE RE-CHALLENGES If your symptoms return when you reintroduce gluten, you may decide to follow a gluten-free diet. If you take this route, consider doing periodic re-challenge tests. It's possible your sensitivity to gluten may be temporary. While you may not be able to eat foods containing gluten right now, that doesn't necessarily mean you'll never be able to eat them. In the future, your body may become more tolerant to gluten and you won't experience symptoms or they may be less severe.

Finding a healthy balance

A primary reason for doing an elimination and re-challenge diet is to take some of the guesswork out of your condition. Of course, it would be better if you could simply take a test to identify if gluten — or some other substance — is the culprit behind your discomfort. Researchers are working on such a test that will hopefully be available in the future. But for right now it's a slow and sometimes lengthy process.

Based on the results of an elimination diet, you may conclude that you have NCGS or, perhaps, sensitivity to another substance in food, such as FODMAPs.

Researchers studying gluten and wheat disorders are questioning if gluten and wheat are just part of the problem. They believe other food components may be to blame for signs and symptoms generally attributed to NCGS. One area of research is a group of carbohydrates that don't digest easily in the small intestine and that ferment or cause bacterial growth when they reach the large intestine. People who are sensitive to these carbohydrates may experience excessive gas, bloating, cramps and diarrhea, similar to NCGS.

The scientific name for these carbohydrates is fermentable oligosaccharides, disaccharides, monosaccharides and polyols (FODMAPs*). For your purposes, it's enough to know the different kinds of FODMAPs and some of the foods that contain high amounts of them:

→ **Fructose.** It's found in high-fructose corn syrup, honey, apples, pears, asparagus and artichokes, as well as other vegetables and fruits.
→ **Lactose.** It's present in milk, yogurt, ice cream and other dairy products.
→ **Oligosaccharides (fructans and galactans).** They're present in wheat, rye, chickpeas, lentils, red kidney beans, garlic, onions, broccoli, watermelon and other vegetables and fruits.
→ **Polyols.** They're found in fruits and vegetables such as apples, plums, peaches, avocados, mushrooms and cauliflower, and reduced-calorie sweeteners known as sugar alcohols.

Following a diet low in FODMAPs is sometimes recommended to treat irritable bowel syndrome (IBS) and other digestive disorders. It doesn't cure IBS, but it may prevent the need for medications.

In one study, people who benefitted from a gluten-free diet were later placed on a different diet in which all foods containing FODMAPs were removed from their diet, in addition to all foods containing gluten. When gluten was introduced back into their diet, these individuals didn't experience any symptoms. This suggests their symptoms weren't due to gluten but perhaps to FODMAPs.

Based on these findings, some researchers began to question if components of wheat other than gluten — such as fructans — could be wholly or partially responsible for symptoms previously attributed to NCGS. Also, how do FODMAPs figure into an elimination diet? Do some people's symptoms improve because gluten is eliminated or because a number of FODMAPs have been removed from the diet? There's much more to learn.

*FODMAP is a trademark of P.R. Gibson and S.J. Shepherd, Monash University, Victoria, Australia.

With either condition, it's important to find a healthy balance — a balance between blaming food for your symptoms and recognizing that other factors also can cause them. Symptoms often associated with food sensitivities can also result from stress, anxiety and depression. Your discomfort may not be solely linked to the food you eat but to other factors in your life as well.

Unfortunately, in an ongoing desire to feel better, some people keep eliminating more and more food from their diets, thinking food is to blame. This can lead to serious malnutrition as well as excessive anxiety about their health that can result in other health issues. Constantly worrying or obsessing about food also can make you miserable and your family miserable. The key for many people who may have NCGS or another type of sensitivity is to find a healthy balance to life. This means taking part in healthy activities, such as daily exercise, meditation and other relaxation techniques, in addition to watching what you eat.

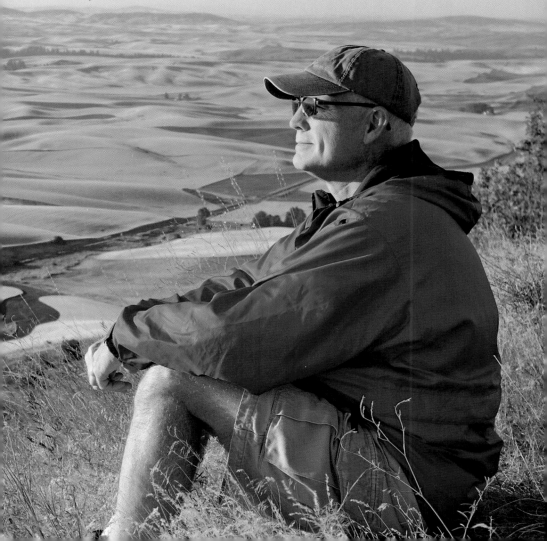

CHAPTER TEN

Other wheat-related disorders

Gluten found in wheat, barley and rye is clearly responsible for a wide variety of symptoms in an increasing number of people. However, there are other components in wheat that can cause trouble, too. There are also various ways that wheat can produce an adverse reaction within the body.

These differences matter. If you think your symptoms are related specifically to foods made from wheat, it's important to work with a doctor or dietitian to pinpoint the exact culprit and the exact mechanism of your reaction. This chapter will help you understand other wheat-related disorders, which can help you get the right diagnosis and treatment.

Wheat sensitivity

When you picture all of the gluten- and wheat-related conditions lined up in a row, you'll find celiac disease on one end and wheat allergy on the other (see the illustration on page 117). As you learned in the first part of this book, celiac disease is a well-understood autoimmune reaction triggered by eating gluten. Wheat allergy is often confused with celiac disease, but it's an entirely different and more rare condition. Wheat allergy results from an allergic reaction — not an autoimmune reaction — to proteins found in wheat. You'll learn more about wheat allergy a little later in this chapter.

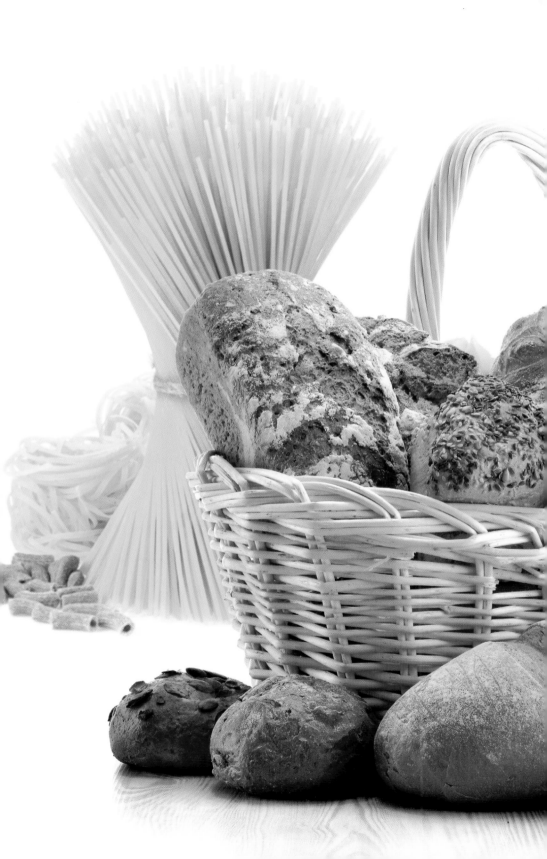

Between these two clear-cut conditions that anchor each end of the spectrum exists a murky middle ground. This is where you find non-celiac gluten sensitivity (NCGS), which was discussed in detail in the last chapter. As you read, researchers are still working to understand this condition. NCGS typically describes individuals who experience symptoms similar to those of celiac disease when they eat food that contains gluten but who don't have specific antibodies or intestinal damage associated with the disease.

What's unclear to researchers is if gluten is always the problem. It's possible that some people who claim to be sensitive to gluten may actually be sensitive to other components of wheat, or to specific substances found in a variety of foods including wheat. For this reason, the term *wheat sensitivity* is sometimes used instead of *gluten sensitivity* to describe symptoms that are similar to NCGS but whose characteristics may be a little different. For instance, an individual may experience uncomfortable symptoms when eating bread made from wheat but not when consuming other products that contain gluten, such as beer or malt vinegar, which get their gluten from barley.

Adding to the confusion, the term *wheat sensitivity* has a variety of meanings. It's sometimes used as an umbrella term to describe any problem related to consuming wheat — including celiac disease, wheat allergy and everything in between. More often, though, it's used to describe a unique condition in which an individual experiences specific signs and symptoms — often gastrointestinal problems such as bloating, gas and diarrhea — after eating products made from wheat. Some people with wheat sensitivity may have other food sensitivities as well.

There are more questions than answers when it comes to wheat sensitivity. Researchers are working to put all of the puzzle pieces together, but the process takes time. What many doctors will agree on at this point is that there's an unclear middle ground between celiac disease and wheat allergy. Conditions that fall into this middle ground appear to result from a reaction to eating wheat or gluten that's neither an autoimmune reaction nor an allergic reaction. The tricky part is that symptoms of various gluten- and wheat-related conditions are similar. Distinguishing the specific cause of the problem can be difficult, and it often takes time.

The work of discerning your exact spot along the line of gluten- and wheat-related conditions is important. There's no reason to follow a more restrictive diet than you need to. For example, you shouldn't assume that you're sensitive to all forms of gluten just because you experience some symptoms when you eat bread and pasta. You may be able to safely eat barley or rye, which means your diet wouldn't have to be as limited.

In addition, the long-term consequences and possible complications vary with the various disorders. The bottom line is, if you're having problems see your doctor. If you haven't been tested for celiac disease, that should be your first step. In order to determine what you do have, it's important to know what you don't have. With the help of your doctor and a dietitian, you may be able to get a better grasp of your condition and better understand what you can and can't eat.

Wheat allergy

Wheat allergy is an allergic reaction to foods that contain wheat. It's one of the more common food allergies in children; however, many children outgrow the allergy before reaching adulthood.

Wheat allergy isn't the same as celiac disease, non-celiac gluten sensitivity or wheat sensitivity. The trigger — wheat — may be the source of all of these conditions, but the body's response to wheat and the best course of treatment are different.

Is it safe to eat wheatgrass?

Wheatgrass is a nutrient-rich type of young grass in the wheat family. It's sold as a dietary supplement in tablet, capsule and liquid forms. Wheatgrass is often used for juicing or added to smoothies or tea. Proponents say that wheatgrass has numerous health benefits, but there are no significant research studies to support these claims.

Wheatgrass, in its pure form, is considered safe for people with celiac disease because it's made from just the grass of the wheat plant and it doesn't contain any seeds. Gluten is found in the seeds. While wheatgrass itself is gluten-free, it matters how the grass is harvested and processed to prevent cross-contamination with grains containing gluten. Products made from wheatgrass can carry a gluten-free label, as long as they contain less than 20 parts per million of gluten.

As for individuals with wheat allergy, it's probably best to avoid products that contain wheatgrass. Wheatgrass has been shown to produce allergic reactions in some people including rashes, throat swelling and breathing difficulty.

To be on the safe side, if you have questions about wheatgrass, check with your doctor before taking anything with wheatgrass in it.

In the case of wheat allergy, your body's immune system mistakenly identifies the proteins found in wheat as harmful intruders. It reacts by producing an allergy-causing antibody called immunoglobulin E. There are four different classes of proteins in wheat that can cause allergies: albumin, globulin, gliadin and gluten. Any of them can produce an allergic reaction. In contrast, in celiac disease, one particular protein in wheat — gluten — causes an abnormal immune system reaction, which damages the small intestine.

SYMPTOMS If you have wheat allergy, you'll likely experience a reaction a few minutes to a few hours after eating food containing wheat. Similar to other food allergies, wheat allergy commonly causes these signs and symptoms:

- Hives or skin rash
- Swelling, itching or irritation of the lips or tongue, and sometimes other parts of the body
- Difficulty breathing or asthma
- Stomach cramps or indigestion
- Nausea or vomiting
- Diarrhea

Symptoms may range from mild to severe. If your response to wheat tends to manifest itself in gastrointestinal signs and symptoms — such as stomach cramps, indigestion or diarrhea — you may think that you have celiac disease or non-celiac gluten sensitivity. Because it's nearly impossible to tell the difference through symptoms alone, it's important to see a doctor for testing. It's rare, however, for wheat allergy to cause only gastrointestinal symptoms without other signs and symptoms, such as hives and itching.

For some people, wheat allergy can also produce a life-threatening reaction called anaphylaxis. Anaphylaxis may cause:

- Swelling or tightness of the throat
- Chest pain or tightness
- Severe difficulty breathing
- Trouble swallowing
- Pale blue skin color
- Dizziness or fainting
- Fast heartbeat

This severe allergic reaction starts rapidly and can be deadly, if not treated promptly with medication.

DIAGNOSIS There are several different ways your doctor can determine if you're allergic to wheat. The route you take will depend on the symptoms that you experience. You may start with a trip to your primary care doctor, who may refer you to a specialist for testing and diagnosis. If your main problems are stomach problems and diarrhea, you may be referred to a gastroenterologist. In contrast, if you tend to experience hives, swelling, runny nose and itchy eyes, you may be referred to an allergist.

The specialist you see will likely conduct a physical examination and ask a lot of questions about your symptoms, your family's history of allergy and asthma, medications you take, and the circumstances surrounding your symptoms. He or she will use this information to help determine the best tests and diagnostic tools to pinpoint the cause of your reaction. Wheat allergy can be difficult to diagnose because wheat is a common food ingredient that may be eaten at many meals along with many other foods.

The following tests can be helpful in diagnosing wheat allergy.

Skin test Skin prick testing is one of the most common tests used in the evaluation of food allergies. It's very effective in determining which allergens are responsible for your reactions so that you can avoid them in the future. Skin prick testing is typically performed under the guidance of a trained allergy specialist who is prepared to treat any severe allergic reactions that may occur.

In a skin prick test, a nurse or doctor applies tiny drops of suspected allergens — such as milk, peanuts, tree nuts, soy, shellfish and wheat — to your skin. Then he or she pricks through the allergens into the top layer of skin. This is usually done on your forearm, but it may be done on your upper back. Many suspected allergens can be tested at the same time.

If you're allergic to wheat, within 15 minutes you'll develop a red, itchy bump — sort of like a mosquito bite — at the spot where the wheat allergen was pricked into your skin. If you're allergic to other allergens, your arm may look like it was bitten by a swarm of mosquitos. However, the effect is only temporary. Severe reactions during skin testing are rare.

This test may not be recommended if you have a history of severe allergic reactions, asthma, or a widespread skin condition, such as dermatitis or psoriasis, which may make it difficult to interpret your reactions. Certain medications, such as antihistamines, steroids and some antidepressants, may also interfere with skin testing.

Blood test An allergy blood test identifies food allergies by provoking an allergic reaction in a test tube, rather than on your arm. For this test, a sample of blood is taken from a vein in your arm and sent to a laboratory where it's combined with allergen proteins. Lab technicians look for signs of specific allergy-causing antibodies called immunoglobulin E (IgE), which your body produces when it's having an allergic response.

Wheat-dependent, exercise-induced anaphylaxis (WDEIA) and baker's asthma are two distinct forms of wheat allergy that occur within specific environments. Another rare condition possibly involving wheat also is under study.

WDEIA. Some people with a wheat allergy develop symptoms only when they exercise within a few hours after eating wheat. Symptoms may begin at any time during exercise, and they can be severe. Typical signs and symptoms include warmth or flushing, rash, large hives, sudden fatigue, nausea, and abdominal cramping. The symptoms usually improve immediately when exercise is stopped.

Unfortunately, some people don't realize the seriousness of their symptoms. Instead, they keep pushing and gasping their way through their workouts. Others run for help, which can dramatically worsen their symptoms. Continued exertion can cause symptoms to progress to wheezing, swelling of the hands and face, difficulty breathing, and even passing out.

Vigorous forms of exercise — such as jogging, aerobics and racket sports — are the most common triggers of this condition, but even less vigorous forms of exercise, including brisk walking or yardwork can trigger it. People with this type of allergy can usually eat wheat without experiencing any symptoms, as long as they don't exercise for a specific period of time afterward. It's the combination of the two that triggers an attack.

Blood testing is more expensive than skin prick testing and it takes more time to complete — unlike skin prick testing, which can give results in about 15 minutes. However, blood testing is a good alternative if skin prick testing is not an option for you. It may also be combined with other tests.

Food diary Sometimes it can be hard to pinpoint which foods you're allergic to, and it's possible that you may be allergic to several foods. Keeping a detailed record of the foods that you eat and the symptoms that you experience can be helpful. A written record can help identify patterns in your reactions, as well as point out foods that you never suspected might be causing your problems.

Your doctor may ask you to keep a thorough food log for a couple of weeks to help answer these questions: How soon after eating do symptoms appear? Do symptoms seem to be related to a specific food? How much of a suspect-

Some people experience an attack only if other triggers are present in addition to exercise and wheat — such as extreme heat and humidity or high pollen levels. Drinking alcoholic beverages or taking nonsteroidal anti-inflammatory drugs (NSAIDs) can also be a contributing factor. There are many different theories about exactly why this occurs. It's also possible that foods other than wheat may trigger symptoms.

Baker's asthma. Baker's asthma is an allergic reaction to certain proteins in wheat flour, rye flour and barley flour. However, this type of allergic reaction is triggered by inhaling the flour, rather than eating it. As the name of this condition implies, baker's asthma is an occupational hazard for bakers, millers, pastry factory workers or anyone who works with uncooked flour. It typically causes problems with breathing. People with baker's asthma can usually eat cooked wheat products without having a reaction.

Eosinophilic esophagitis. This recently recognized condition is still under study. It's characterized by inflammation and narrowing of the esophagus, causing food to get held up in the esophagus. The condition predominantly affects males but may also affect females. It often occurs in individuals with allergic disorders, and may be more common in people with celiac disease. Some information suggests wheat and milk may be triggers for the condition.

ed allergy-causing food was eaten? What other foods were eaten at or around the same time as the food you suspect is causing your symptoms?

Elimination diet Your doctor may recommend that you remove certain foods from your diet to see if this affects your symptoms. Under your doctor's direction, you may gradually add foods back into your diet and note if and when your symptoms return. See page 130 for more information on an elimination diet.

Food challenge A food challenge is a carefully structured program in which you eat foods suspected of causing your allergies under the close supervision of a trained specialist. A food challenge usually follows an elimination diet, and it takes place in a hospital or clinic. Often, you can't tell what foods you're eating during a food challenge, so the results are unbiased.

Your doctor may recommend a food challenge if he or she suspects a particular food is responsible for your reactions but allergy blood tests or skin tests for this food, or both, are negative. You may also undergo a food challenge if avoiding suspected allergens hasn't resolved your symptoms and further evidence is needed to guide your treatment plan. Some people also undergo a food challenge to determine if they have outgrown a food allergy. You should never try a food challenge on your own at home.

Exercise challenge If your doctor believes that you have a condition known as wheat-dependent, exercise-induced anaphylaxis (WDEIA), you may undergo an exercise challenge under close supervision to confirm this diagnosis. For more information on WDEIA, see page 140.

TREATMENT The best treatment for wheat allergy is strict avoidance of anything that contains wheat protein. Even the tiniest amount can cause an allergic reaction in some people.

This can be difficult because many different food products contain some form of wheat. Some sources of wheat are obvious, such as bread, breadcrumbs, cookies, cereal, crackers and pasta. But this grain and its derivatives are hidden in some unexpected places, including hot dogs, candy, salad dressings, soups and soy sauce. The next section of this book provides you with tips on how to avoid wheat in your diet. You'll also find ideas for incorporating wheat-free grains and ingredients into your meals.

Some people who are allergic to wheat are also allergic to other grains with similar proteins, such as barley, rye and oats. If this is your situation, you may need to adopt a gluten-free diet, also described in the next part of this book. On the other hand, if you're allergic only to wheat, you may not need to give up all foods that contain gluten, just those made from wheat.

A gluten-free diet is usually safe for someone who is allergic to wheat, because it generally doesn't contain any wheat. But it's still important to check the ingredients. In some countries, foods may contain ingredients made from wheat starch in which most of the gluten has been removed. These foods may be labeled gluten-free yet still contain wheat. If they do, the label should say the product contains wheat. If the label doesn't say that the food contains wheat, it should be safe to eat.

A gluten-free diet, however, may be more limiting than you need. Work with your doctor to understand all of the foods that you need to avoid, and then read the next section of this book carefully. Zero in on the information that's relevant to you. You want to eliminate those foods that you can't tolerate.

If you have wheat-dependent exercise-induced anaphylaxis (WDEIA) or baker's asthma, you may be able to eat some foods that contain wheat. But you'll need to be careful to avoid a severe allergic reaction. Work with your doctor to make sure that you understand how to take care of yourself and how to avoid triggering an attack.

MEDICATIONS Despite your best attempts to avoid wheat, you may unknowingly eat something that contains wheat — at a restaurant, a party or even in your own home. It's important to be prepared to treat an unexpected allergic reaction. To do so, your doctor may prescribe the following medications.

Antihistamines These oral medications may reduce some signs and symptoms of wheat allergy, such as itching and hives. You can take this medication as soon as you experience symptoms or if you believe you just ate something that contains wheat. Antihistamines can help control your reaction and relieve discomfort. They're available over-the-counter and by prescription.

Just remember that antihistamines aren't meant to treat dangerous allergic symptoms, such as throat swelling and difficulty breathing. Their response time is slower. They're not rapid enough for an emergency situation.

Epinephrine Epinephrine can reverse the dangerous symptoms associated with a severe allergic reaction. If you're at risk of having a severe reaction to wheat, you may need to carry an epinephrine auto-injector (EpiPen, Auvi-Q) with you at all times in case an emergency should arise. Each auto-injector contains one dose of medication that can be injected into your thigh. Your doctor or a medical professional can teach you and your loved ones how to use this medication. Epinephrine is intended to help control a severe allergic reaction until emergency medical care arrives.

Epinephrine works best when given within the first few minutes of a severe allergic reaction. Don't hesitate to use it if you have trouble breathing or you have tightness in your throat. This medication can save your life. After receiving the medication, it's still important to get emergency medical help. Epinephrine can wear off in 15 to 30 minutes, and the symptoms could return.

Keep others informed of your wheat allergy, and make sure they know how to help in case of an emergency.

How to eat without wheat

Living with an allergy or sensitivity to wheat can be challenging. You need to be vigilant about everything that you eat — at home, at work and everywhere you go. Over time, though, the task becomes easier. The information in the next section of this book can help you learn how to live and eat well, despite needing to steer clear of all things wheat.

CHAPTER ELEVEN

Choosing to go gluten-free

Eating often isn't an enjoyable experience for Tom. Shortly after finishing a meal, he gets a headache and feels tired. Sometimes he has trouble concentrating, with the sensation that his brain is "foggy." Tom believes that gluten may be the problem — his body doesn't react well to it. He was tested for celiac disease and the results came back negative. Still, Tom is considering trying out a gluten-free diet. Maybe he doesn't have celiac disease, but could he be sensitive to gluten? Tom wonders, though, if he can stay on the diet. His mother is Italian, and Tom can't imagine life without her gluten-loaded pasta dinners.

Then there's Jennifer. She's an avid runner and has just signed up for a 5K race. She's trying to eat as "clean" as possible to improve her performance. A girlfriend introduced her to several gluten-free recipes, and these foods have become some of her favorites. Now, Jennifer is thinking about giving up gluten entirely. She doesn't have celiac disease and she isn't gluten sensitive, but she's heard that eating gluten-free is healthy. She believes eliminating gluten will help her eat better and feel more energetic. Plus, she heard that getting rid of gluten might reduce her migraines.

Is your situation similar to either of these? Whether you're like Tom, who wonders if he can eat gluten-free, or like Jennifer, who fully embraces this change, there are important things to know before you make the switch.

This chapter introduces key factors that can help guide your decision about whether to follow a gluten-free diet. The chapter also highlights steps to ensure you maintain good health if you do decide to eliminate gluten.

As you work your way through this chapter, it may seem like there's a lot to take in. Fully understanding the positives and negatives of a gluten-free eating plan can help you decide if this type of diet is for you. Being aware of the hurdles that lie ahead also can help ease the transition to gluten freedom.

The chapters in the next section of this book provide plenty of practical tips, shortcuts and strategies to assist you. Keep in mind that the longer you follow a gluten-free diet, the simpler and easier it becomes. You'll find that some foods you've been eating may already be gluten-free and that there are many new gluten-free foods ready to explore.

If you have celiac disease, there's no choice to be made about going gluten-free. You need to eliminate gluten from your diet to manage the disease and stay healthy. In a sense, this chapter doesn't apply to you because the decision about whether to eat gluten-free has already been made. However, the chapter contains some valuable information, so it may be worth your time to read on.

Are there positives to a gluten-free diet?

The benefits of avoiding gluten are being touted everywhere — in best-selling books and popular magazines, on websites and TV news programs. What began as a treatment for celiac disease has become a trendy worldwide food phenomenon. If you believe everything you read in the popular media, you might think a gluten-free diet is a surefire way to lose weight, boost energy, improve performance and reach maximum health. The truth is, it's a big stretch to accomplish most, if any, of that.

For celiac disease, the benefit of a gluten-free diet is clear. Ridding your body of gluten will allow your small intestine to heal so that it and the rest of your body can operate normally again. Your symptoms should disappear and those organs once deprived of vital nourishment should return to good health. Sticking to a gluten-free diet for the rest of your life is essential. It's the only way to treat celiac disease.

For other gluten-related disorders, such as non-celiac gluten sensitivity, a gluten-free diet may also be an effective treatment. As you read in previous chapters, there's much that isn't known when it comes to gluten-related conditions other than celiac disease. However, many people who believe they're sensitive to gluten find they feel better when they remove gluten from their diets. This may be because they're no longer eating gluten. Or it could be because they're no longer eating other ingredients that are common to foods that contain gluten.

Will eating gluten-free help me lose weight? The answer is, it depends.

Some people with celiac disease unintentionally lose weight before they're diagnosed with the disease because their small intestine can't absorb the vital nutrients from food, causing these individuals to experience malnutrition. As their condition improves, these individuals typically regain weight.

For some others, the opposite may be true. Some people who follow a gluten-free diet lose some weight. Typically, the reason why is because they're eating healthier than before they went gluten-free. They're eating fewer processed foods and more natural, whole foods. And by doing so, they're consuming fewer calories. It's the reduction in calories that's responsible for the drop in weight, not the elimination of gluten from their diets.

Whether you gain or lose weight on a gluten-free diet is generally dependent on your overall health when you start the diet and the foods you eat. Just because a product is labeled gluten-free doesn't mean it's healthy for you. Sometimes it may contain even more fat and calories than its gluten-filled counterpart. And if you're swapping a regular cookie for handfuls of gluten-free but calorie-filled cookies, you're likely to gain weight.

The best way to lose unwanted pounds is to change your eating and exercise habits. This principle applies to all types of diets, not just a gluten-free diet.

Can a gluten-free diet help cure other common diseases? Researchers have investigated the merits of a gluten-free diet for dozens of conditions, including irritable bowel syndrome, rheumatoid arthritis, autism, psoriasis, multiple sclerosis, migraines, thyroid disease and diabetes, with varying results. Based on the strength of the evidence so far, most doctors don't recommend going gluten-free if you don't have a gluten-related condition.

However, if you feel that eliminating gluten will help you feel better and the diet won't interfere with treatment for other conditions you may have, there's probably no harm in giving it a try, as long as you eat healthy. It's a good idea, though, to discuss this change with your doctor. He or she may want to check you for celiac disease beforehand (see page 156).

KEEP IT HEALTHY Similar to any good meal plan, the way to eat healthy when following a gluten-free diet is to consume a mixture of foods from the major food groups, and to keep your proportions in check. You want to replace foods that contain gluten with healthy alternatives.

A gluten-free diet often forces people to give up processed foods in favor of an unprocessed diet. In this respect, the diet can be good for you. If instead of eating crackers, sugary breakfast cereals, desserts and pastries, you find yourself eating more natural foods, such as fruits, vegetables, meat and cheese, then your health is likely to benefit.

If, however, you simply swap a regular cracker or cookie for a gluten-free version, there's no benefit from that. You're not eating any better than when you were eating foods that contained gluten. In fact, some gluten-free foods are worse for you than their regular counterparts because they contain more sugar, fat and sodium and less fiber.

So, how you approach the diet is key. If you go gluten-free with the goal of reducing the amount of processed foods you eat in favor of more natural foods, you're on the right path.

Drawbacks of eating gluten-free

As with most things in life, not everything about eating gluten-free is easy. There are definite downsides to the diet. Some problems involve certain nutrient deficiencies. When you adopt a gluten-free diet, you're giving up many foods with important nutritional value. For example, regular bread and pasta are often nutrient fortified, and foods made from whole wheat are often good sources of antioxidants and fiber, which can reduce your risks of many major illnesses. You'll want to find ways to replace these lost nutrients.

LESS FIBER Fiber is probably best known for its ability to prevent and relieve constipation — for good reason. Dietary fiber helps to bulk up and soften your stools, making it easier to pass them. Beyond bowel health, a high-fiber diet may also lower cholesterol, help control blood sugar levels and help you maintain a healthy weight.

In the United States, wheat is a major source of dietary fiber. When you take wheat out of your diet, you may eliminate much of your recommended daily intake of fiber as well. This can lead to constipation and stomach cramps.

Thankfully, fiber is also found in many gluten-free foods. This includes vegetables, fruits, nuts and seeds, and gluten-free whole grains, such as quinoa, brown rice and gluten-free oats. Beans, peas and other legumes are also excellent, inexpensive sources of fiber.

An important part of going gluten-free involves making sure your diet contains enough fiber. You want to eat plenty of fruits and vegetables each day, and include whole grains that don't contain gluten. Fiber-rich snacks

How much fiber do you need?

	Age 50 or younger	Age 51 or older
Men	38 grams	30 grams
Women	25 grams	21 grams

Source: Institute of Medicine

include popcorn, dried fruits, carrots and nuts. And be sure to eat fruits that still have their fiber-rich skins on, such as apples.

FEWER FRUCTANS Wheat, barley and rye also contain fructans. Fructan is a type of carbohydrate that provides food for healthy bacteria in the colon, called probiotics. Wheat is the biggest source of fructans in the food supply. When you eliminate wheat from your diet, you also eliminate this source of healthy bacteria.

REDUCED VITAMINS AND MINERALS Most people don't think much about vitamins and minerals until they experience the health consequences of not getting enough of them. Regular wheat bread, as well as cereal and pasta products made with wheat, are often enriched or fortified with vitamins and minerals during processing. If you're no longer eating these foods, you may not be getting enough of certain key nutrients. Serious consequences of a vitamin and mineral deficiency may include anemia, impaired immunity, birth defects, learning problems and memory loss.

Currently, enrichment and fortification practices aren't commonplace in most specially prepared gluten-free products. So if you eat a lot of gluten-free substitutes, you may be losing a major source of vitamins and minerals.

Concern about reduced vitamins and minerals could change as the demand for gluten-free products increases and more large-volume food manufacturers get into the gluten-free game. Some enriched and fortified gluten-free products are already available, and before long, there may be a wider selection of healthy options. For now, though, it's important to pay attention to certain vitamins and minerals that are difficult to include in a gluten-free diet. These include:

B vitamins The B vitamins, which include thiamin, riboflavin, niacin and folate, can be found in many vegetables, fruits, meat, fish, dairy products and legumes. B vitamins help maintain nerve cells and red blood cells. Low levels of some of

Enriched vs. fortified

These two labels commonly found on foods aren't synonymous. Understanding the terms may help you decide which food products you should buy.

Enriched. This means that some of the nutrients lost during the milling process are added back in. You'll see this label on products that use refined grains, such as white bread, white flour, breakfast cereals and regular pasta.

Refined grains are milled, a process that strips out both the bran and germ to give the grains a finer texture. The refining process also removes many nutrients, including fiber. When foods are enriched, some of these lost vitamins — such as thiamin, niacin and riboflavin (some of the B vitamins), for instance — are added back in.

Fortified. Fortifying a food means adding in nutrients that aren't naturally found in the food. Many enriched foods are fortified with additional vitamins and minerals, such as folic acid and iron.

For example, fortified foods are an important source of vitamin D in the United States. Almost all of the milk in the United States is voluntarily fortified with vitamin D as the result of a public health initiative. Ready-to-eat breakfast cereals and other grain products are fortified with folic acid and iron as well as vitamin D.

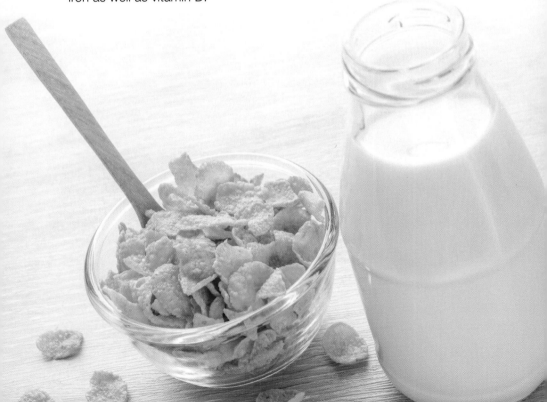

these vitamins may be linked to memory loss and depression. In addition, folate is a B vitamin that's important for preventing serious birth defects. Adequate folate is essential if you're planning to get pregnant or are already pregnant.

Calcium Your body needs an adequate supply of calcium to build and maintain strong bones. Your heart, muscles and nerves also need calcium to function properly. A gluten-free diet is not inherently low in calcium, but if the amount you consume is limited, perhaps because of lactose intolerance, you need to be sure to get adequate calcium elsewhere. In addition to dairy products, sources of calcium include some legumes, sesame seeds, nuts, oranges and dark green leafy vegetables, such as kale and turnip greens.

Vitamin D This vitamin is essential for helping your body absorb calcium and maintain optimal bone health. Vitamin D is produced in the skin in response to sunlight, but if you live in a northern climate or stay out of the sun to protect your skin, your dominant source of the vitamin is from food.

Similar to calcium, a gluten-free diet is not inherently low in vitamin D, but you still need adequate amounts of the vitamin to reduce your risk of osteoporosis. If you don't drink milk, you've eliminated certain fortified products by going gluten-free and you don't take a multivitamin, you're likely not getting enough vitamin D. Ask your doctor if you should take a vitamin D supplement and, if so, how much of the supplement.

Iron Your body needs iron to produce hemoglobin. This mineral enables red blood cells to carry oxygenated blood throughout your body. If you're short on iron, you may feel tired and out of breath because oxygen isn't distributed normally. When you give up gluten, you eliminate grain products that are iron fortified. Thankfully, many naturally gluten-free foods, such as lean red meat, beans and lentils, dark green vegetables, and dried fruits and nuts, are sources of iron. Just make sure that you're eating enough of them!

Vitamin and mineral deficiencies can cause serious health complications if not identified and treated. To maintain your health, actively seek out strategies for replacing vitamins and minerals that may be missing following your switch to a gluten-free diet. Your doctor will help you determine if supplements are needed, and your dietitian can help you improve your food choices.

COST AND AVAILABILITY The market for gluten-free foods and beverages has grown by leaps and bounds in the last decade. Today, gluten-free products are a multibillion-dollar business.

This is good news, because it means that gluten-free foods are becoming more widely available. Over time, greater supply and more competition may

ITEM	PRICE
BAKERY	4.50
CEREAL	3.25
OIL	1.95
DELI	6.59
PRODUCE	.89
PRODUCE	2.29
FRUIT	3.67
DRESSING	2.59
BOTTLED WATER	1.99
BATH	1.50
KITCHEN	1.29
PASTA	2.05
TOMATOES	1.15
EGGS	2.59
APPLESAUCE	.99
BUTTER	1.60
BREAD	2.60
RICE	1.30
CRACKERS	2.75
PRODUCE	1.86
YOGURT	1.00
BEANS	1.59
CHEESE	5.53
PUDDING	1.89
CHIPS	1.59
SUBTOTAL	59.00
TAX	.90
TOTAL	59.90

THANK YOU
COME AGAIN

also drive down the costs of these items. But that's not reality yet. Gluten-free foods and beverages are still several times more expensive than their conventional counterparts. This can be a hassle and a financial hardship for some.

In addition to the expense, depending on where you live, gluten-free products may not be available in your local grocery store. In some areas, gluten-free options are scarce or only stocked at specialty stores. Price and inconvenience are factors to consider if you don't have to go gluten-free but are considering doing so. It takes planning and determination to make the diet work.

TIME Starting any diet involves a learning curve — going gluten-free is no exception. Switching to a gluten-free diet may seem complicated. A lot of this has to do with learning a new language — the language of food labels. You need to look for the "gluten-free" label on a package and understand what it means — less than 20 parts per million (ppm) of gluten, which is considered harmless for most people with celiac disease.

You also need to learn what to look for on the ingredient list that accompanies every product. Gluten comes disguised under many names. With time, you'll come to know what does and doesn't contain gluten. But in the beginning, grocery shopping will take more time. Be patient; the time you spend up front will make adapting to the diet easier.

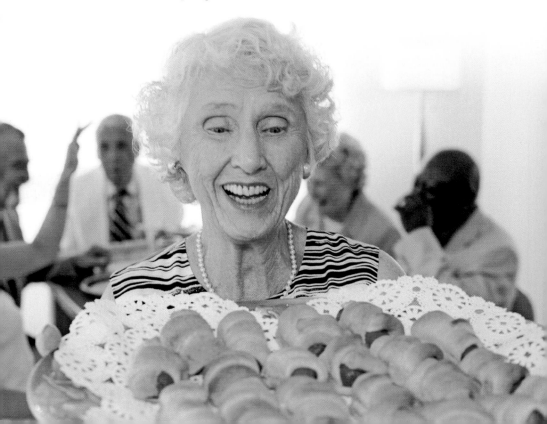

IMPACT ON YOUR FAMILY AND SOCIAL LIFE Adopting a gluten-free diet isn't something that only you have to deal with. This change also affects your family and friends. Some people close to you will take a keen interest and learn quickly. Other people may never ever get it. Your well-meaning aunt may demand that you try her famous gluten-packed Thanksgiving stuffing or her tasty breaded appetizers, despite your protests.

Be prepared that well-intentioned people will mistakenly try to serve you food that contains gluten. These individuals are not trying to derail your diet. They simply may not recognize that so many foods contain gluten, and they don't suspect gluten in many common products.

It's also important to consider how you will manage the diet at home. There are a lot of questions to ask yourself and your family. Will your entire family be eating gluten-free or just you? Is your family up for this change in diet? If you're the only one going gluten-free, what will you do at meal-times? Will you need to prepare two meals? And will your family be willing to go to restaurants that offer gluten-free options? How will you handle social events in which there may not be gluten-free options?

These questions may not have easy answers. The intention is not to steer you away from eating gluten-free. Rather, they're necessary aspects to consider. A gluten-free diet shouldn't separate you from your family or hold you back from a full social calendar. You'll find strategies for eating out and attending parties in this book. You'll also learn about ways to fit a complete gluten-free diet into your busy family life so that you don't have to cook two dinners every night. Meal preparation should be as practical and easy as possible so that you can stick to the diet.

Reduction vs. elimination

For many individuals with non-celiac gluten sensitivity, it's not necessary to get rid of all gluten in order to feel better. This is different from celiac disease, which requires complete elimination of gluten to prevent serious complications. Nor do all people with wheat sensitivity need to avoid wheat to the same extent that individuals with wheat allergy must do.

What this means is that if you're sensitive to gluten or wheat, it may be sufficient to limit your intake to the point that your symptoms disappear and you feel good. You may find that small amounts here and there may be OK.

Options for going gluten-free

As mentioned earlier, if you have celiac disease, there's really no decision to be made. A gluten-free diet is a must. It's important that you completely eliminate all gluten from your diet. If you don't have celiac disease, you have some options.

If you think that you may be sensitive to gluten, you might want to start a gluten-free diet and see how you feel. If you find that your symptoms disappear and you feel better, it may be in your best interests to continue the diet. Some people who claim to be sensitive to gluten find that they can tolerate a small amount of gluten without it bothering them, but they don't need to avoid it entirely. Other people only feel better if all gluten is removed from their diet.

If you have no medical reason to follow a gluten-free diet but you'd like to do so because you think it'll be better for your health, there are different options you can take. One option is to eliminate all gluten from your diet. Another option is to reduce the amount of gluten in your diet. For example, you may avoid gluten at home but choose to eat gluten occasionally at social events, when eating out or at holiday gatherings.

Or you may decide that gluten-free isn't for you. Think about your personal situation, symptoms and health goals, as well as the benefits and shortcomings of the gluten-free diet described in this chapter. If your goal is to eat healthier, there may be other ways to do that, including eating more fruits and vegetables and limiting foods high in sugar, fat and sodium.

Also, consider how long you intend to stick to this diet. A few weeks? A few months? A lifetime? The time it takes to become proficient with eating gluten-free may not be worth your while if you're just looking for a short-term fix.

See your doctor

It's tempting to jump right onto the gluten-free bandwagon if you're thinking that a gluten-free diet may be the solution to your health problems. But if you're planning to make that leap, the first step you should take is to visit with your doctor. (Actually, consulting your doctor is a good start to any major dietary change you make, whether that change involves gluten or not.)

Your doctor can evaluate your health status and help you decide if a gluten-free diet will be safe and effective, based on your personal history and on your health goals. Your doctor can also provide general dietary advice to make sure that you're getting adequate fiber, vitamins and minerals. For example, you may need to pay particular attention to certain nutrients if you're taking medications, planning to get pregnant, or have a history of osteoporosis and bone loss or other conditions.

It's especially important to talk to your doctor or a dietitian before you adopt a gluten-free diet if you're already following a special diet for other health conditions, such as high blood pressure or diabetes. In this case, all of your specialized dietary needs will need to be addressed — carbohydrate control (diabetes), lower sodium (high blood pressure) — in addition to eliminating gluten.

Your doctor also can determine if you should undergo celiac testing before you go gluten-free. If you have no symptoms or risk factors for celiac disease, your doctor may not recommend the test. But if you have a family history of celiac disease or you're exhibiting symptoms of the condition, your doctor may schedule a celiac test before you start a gluten-free diet.

If you begin a gluten-free diet before being tested for celiac disease, the test may produce a false-negative result — indicating that you don't have celiac disease when you really do. For an accurate result, you will need to go back on a regular diet that contains gluten so that there's an adequate amount in your body to trigger the immune reaction. In some cases, you may need to reintroduce gluten under the supervision of your doctor.

In addition, going gluten-free before being tested for celiac disease may delay the diagnosis of another condition. There are many reasons that a gluten-free diet may cause you to feel better. For example, you may notice your bloating and abdominal discomfort have eased since you started the diet. But staying away from gluten may not be the reason. It may be that you're now eating fewer processed foods that contain other ingredients that were triggering your symptoms or that you're eating slower or consuming smaller proportions.

Furthermore, your relief may only be temporary, and may be masking another underlying problem, such as Crohn's disease, colitis, fructose intolerance and a host of other disorders. If you spend months experimenting with a gluten-free diet, convinced that gluten is your problem, you could be delaying the diagnosis and treatment of what's really ailing you.

If you've been eating gluten-free for a while and your symptoms have returned or they never went away, gluten may not be the culprit. But only if you're tested for celiac disease will you know for sure. How to test for celiac disease in people who are already eating gluten-free is discussed on page 72.

It's a personal decision

Gluten is grabbing a lot of attention right now, and it's easy to get caught up in the anti-gluten frenzy. Is it in your best interests to go gluten-free if there's no medical need to do so?

The case for celiac testing

You may wonder, why bother checking with your doctor before you ditch gluten? Do you really need an official medical evaluation to change your diet? The answer is yes, especially if you have symptoms that could possibly be linked to celiac disease. If it turns out that your symptoms are, in fact, due to celiac disease:

You need medical care. Celiac disease inflames and damages the lining of the small intestine, preventing the absorption of some nutrients. It's important to know if you have celiac disease so that you can receive on-going care and monitoring under the guidance of a gastroenterologist and a dietitian who can help you plan a healthy gluten-free diet and manage any problems caused by the disease.

Regular follow-up appointments can confirm that your intestine is healing and that you're getting proper nutrition. Simply switching to a gluten-free diet on your own can't provide that.

Your family members need to be tested. Celiac disease commonly occurs in family members, and it can have serious consequences when not identified and treated. Even if your family members aren't having symptoms, the disease may be causing intestinal damage. If you have the condition, it's important for family members to also be tested and, if necessary, treated.

You'll need to avoid all gluten. Sometimes, when people say they're "gluten-free," they're really eating less gluten. Or they're eating gluten-free except for when they want a piece of birthday cake or a beer, or they have a craving for their favorite meal at the local Italian restaurant.

This lax approach is fine if you don't have celiac disease and you're choosing to avoid gluten for other reasons. But it's not fine if gluten is damaging your small intestine. If you have celiac disease, there are no cheat days. Even trace amounts of gluten can cause serious complications. So you need to be savvy about hidden sources of gluten and cross-contamination in your own kitchen or at restaurants.

If your test results for celiac disease turn out negative, that's still good to know. You know that the disease isn't the cause of your symptoms. Crossing celiac disease off the list may lead you to think differently about your symptoms and what's triggering them.

The best way to answer that question is by stepping back from all the hype and closely examining your personal needs and goals. You don't want to go gluten-free just because it seems like everyone else is doing so. You don't want to make the change because a friend says you should. And you don't want to eliminate gluten because you heard an ominous report about it on the radio this morning. If you decide to go gluten-free, you want to do it because you've discussed it with your doctor and you believe a gluten-free diet is going to benefit you and make you healthier.

Now that you've read about the pros and cons of a gluten-free diet, consider all of the pluses and minuses. Making an educated decision will improve your chances of success in sticking to the diet. The chapters in Part 3 provide detailed information on how to start living gluten-free.

Living Gluten-Free

(and loving it!)

CHAPTER TWELVE

Gluten-free basics

Enjoying a good meal among good company is one of life's great pleasures. This doesn't have to change just because you can't eat gluten. From gourmet dinner parties to casual backyard barbecues, you can still eat well and have fun. Like many people, you may find a gluten-free diet is a lot about changing your routines. If you always start the day with cereal or toast and always pack a sandwich for lunch, you may have to change those habits. But you may also find the changes are more of a minor tweak than a complete overhaul.

Many people find that foods they thought would be off-limits don't have to be. You just have to find new and creative ways to make them. And don't be surprised if some of what you create is better than what you were eating before!

What's also important when eating gluten-free is that you eat well. You can load up on processed foods and still eat gluten-free, but that's not the best approach. Instead, try to follow a diet that's balanced and that provides all of the nutrients that your body needs for good health.

No doubt, adapting to a gluten-free diet may be frustrating at first. While you only need to eliminate one item from your diet — gluten — that one item is found in thousands of foods and is pervasive in the American diet. That's what makes the task complex.

The upcoming chapters will help you learn how to shop for gluten-free foods, how to modify your favorite recipes to eliminate gluten and how to cook new favorites without gluten. This chapter introduces you to the basic principles of the gluten-free diet. You'll learn which foods contain gluten and which ones don't. You'll also learn how to eat healthy on a gluten-free diet and why that's important.

With time and creativity, you'll find that a gluten-free diet doesn't have to stop you from savoring mouthwatering meals with the people that you love and enjoy the most. And take heart in knowing that there's never been a better time to go gluten-free. The number of gluten-free products and meal offerings continues to grow.

Before you begin

As with most new endeavors, it's important to have some strategies in mind before you get started to help you achieve your goals. The same it true for changing your diet. Take a moment to review some key concepts that will help you be successful.

STRATEGY CHECKLIST The following strategies can help make the transition to a gluten-free diet less difficult. Keep them in mind as you do your planning and preparation. More details about these strategies are provided in other parts of the book.

- **Know your goals.** Why are you eliminating gluten? Because you have to, or because you want to? If you have celiac disease, a gluten-free diet is a must. You need to eliminate all gluten to heal your body. If you don't have celiac disease, avoiding gluten may help you feel better; however, you may be able to tolerate small amounts.

- **Look for support.** Don't try to do everything on your own. A doctor and a dietitian can be valuable resources. You might also look for a celiac disease support group in your community (see pages 274 and 275).

- **Eat simple at first.** Begin with unprocessed foods that are naturally gluten-free. This includes fresh vegetables and fruits, poultry, fish, lean meat, rice, potatoes, nuts, and most dairy products. The bulk of your diet may be gluten-free already.

- **Gradually broaden your diet.** As you feel more confident in the changes you're making, expand the selection of foods you eat. Make a list of the foods you can't live without and find gluten-free alternatives or look for ways to modify them. Don't be afraid to try less familiar but naturally gluten-free foods.

❀ **Be prepared for missteps.** It will take some time to master a gluten-free diet. Mistakes are inevitable, particularly from cross-contamination. When this happens, don't beat yourself up. Make it a learning opportunity and move on.

❀ **Embrace your new normal.** Instead of viewing your diet as something terrible, embrace it. Look for the positives in the changes you're making, including future good health.

Building blocks of a gluten-free diet

If you feel overwhelmed by your new diet, don't worry you're not alone. The feeling is natural and it's common. At the same time, most people find that it's not as difficult to give up gluten as they first feared. A gluten-free diet doesn't have to include a bizarre mixture of foods. In fact, it doesn't have to look all that different from a regular diet — one that contains gluten.

The first step in going gluten-free is to understand where gluten lurks — which foods contain gluten and which don't. Let's begin with a quick review of the major food groups.

VEGETABLES AND FRUITS Vegetables and fruits are the foundation of any healthy diet. This is especially true for a gluten-free diet. Vegetables and fruits are naturally gluten-free, so you can eat as many of them as you like. The key is to pay attention to how you prepare them. Some herbs, seasonings, dips or sauces may contain gluten. That's where you need to be careful.

Eating more vegetables and fruits will also help replace some of the fiber, vitamins and minerals that can naturally be lost when you eliminate foods with gluten.

Best gluten-free options Basically all fresh and frozen vegetables and fruits are good gluten-free choices. You can eat them without worry. If they're seasoned or marinated, be sure to check the package labels. The same is true for any processed vegetables and fruits, as well as dried fruit and prepared smoothies. Ingredients that are sometimes added to these products can contain hidden amounts of gluten.

During the summer harvest, nothing beats farm-picked tomatoes, peppers and cucumbers. Year-round, you can usually find carrots, green beans, and salad greens such as lettuce and spinach. In the frozen aisle, look for peas, corn and other vegetables without added sauces. Canned vegetables are OK, too.

When it comes to fruit, feel free to bite into fresh apples, bananas, peaches and plums, and slightly more exotic fruits such as mangoes and papayas. Frozen and canned fruits also can be part of a gluten-free diet. Dried fruits are a good source of fiber in place of fiber-rich grains that contain gluten.

GRAINS This is where the red flag goes up. You need to be cautious about eating any grain products. Foods made from wheat, barley and rye contain gluten. And there are a lot of foods made from these grains — bread, pasta and baked goods such as cakes and cookies, just for starters.

In the next chapter, you'll learn what to look for on food labels so you know if the product is made from wheat, barley or rye.

Not all grains are off-limits, though, because not all grains contain gluten. Rice and corn are naturally gluten-free, and despite its name, so is buckwheat. A key part of eating gluten-free is learning which foods contain gluten-free grains and how to cook with gluten-free grains.

Grains are good sources of B vitamins, iron and fiber, so you want to include them in your diet — you just need to make sure to eat the right ones! At the end of this chapter is a list of grains that don't contain gluten. With time, you'll become more familiar with many of these products.

Best gluten-free options Foods made from naturally gluten-free grains include white and brown rice, corn, grits, popcorn, and corn tortillas. You can also purchase gluten-free breads, cereals, pastas and flours that are made from grains that don't contain gluten.

There are plenty of more obscure grains that are naturally gluten-free, including amaranth, buckwheat, sorghum, millet and quinoa. These can be used in place of regular grains when cooking. They can be added to soups and stews and used as alternatives in casseroles and side dishes. You'll learn more about how to prepare these grains in Chapter 15.

MEATS AND OTHER PROTEIN Meat and many other sources of protein — such as fish, eggs, legumes and nuts — are naturally gluten-free. These are foods you can eat, so enjoy.

Lean meat, poultry and other proteins should comprise a portion of your daily diet. Foods containing protein are good sources of iron, B vitamins and minerals. They can make up for the nutrients you aren't getting from standard enriched and fortified grain products. Legumes, which include beans, peas and lentils, are also excellent sources of fiber, iron and B vitamins.

Best gluten-free options Beef, lamb, pork, chicken and turkey are naturally gluten-free. They are all items that can go in your shopping cart. Keep in mind, however, that they contain saturated fat and cholesterol. So watch your portion sizes and focus on lean cuts of meat and skinless chicken. Other sources of protein with less fat and cholesterol are fish, shellfish and legumes.

When shopping, beware that breadings, coatings and marinades on meat, poultry and fish products may contain gluten. That's why it's recommended that you buy plain pieces of fresh or frozen chicken and fish — not the frozen bag of pre-breaded, precooked ones.

Eggs also are good gluten-free options, as are nuts, seeds and legumes. Beware of peanut butter. It may contain additives that contain gluten, so make sure to read the label and verify it's gluten-free.

DAIRY PRODUCTS Dairy products are a bit of a mixed bag. Milk itself is gluten-free. However, when milk is processed into cheese, yogurt or milk-based desserts, ingredients may be added that contain gluten. So, it's important to read the labels carefully and choose your dairy products wisely.

Dairy products are good for you because they're primary sources of calcium, potassium and vitamin D, nutrients your body needs. Getting adequate calcium and vitamin D is especially important to individuals with celiac disease who may be at risk of osteoporosis due to malabsorption. Calcium and vitamin D can help increase bone mass.

Best gluten-free options Milk and cheese are generally good gluten-free options. Don't be afraid to drink your milk. With other dairy products, such as yogurt and ice cream, most of them are gluten-free, but be sure to read the label to make sure the products don't contain added gluten.

Similar to meat and poultry, dairy products contain saturated fat and some cholesterol, so choose low-fat varieties.

A starter kit

These food staples are naturally gluten-free. If you're just beginning a gluten-free diet, here are some basics to get you started as you learn which foods are safe to eat:

- Fresh meats, poultry and fish
- Eggs
- Fruits
- Vegetables
- Rice
- Potatoes
- Milk and cheese
- Beans, seeds and nuts in their natural form

Oats don't contain gluten — they're naturally gluten-free. However, it's not recommended that people on a gluten-free diet eat them. Why is that? There are a couple of reasons.

First, a couple of studies show that in some people with celiac disease a particular protein in oats can trigger an immune response similar to gluten. This is true only for a small group of people, not for everyone.

Second, and of more concern, is the risk of cross-contamination. Oats are often grown in fields that are rotated with other grains, including wheat, barley and rye. The oats may be contaminated during the harvest before they even arrive at the mill. In addition, most mills that process oats also manufacture wheat, which can result in cross-contamination.

With the increased demand for gluten-free products, some companies are going to great lengths to carefully grow, harvest and process oats in a safe, controlled manner. But for now, it's best to proceed with caution.

If you have celiac disease, don't eat oats until your disease is well under control — for at least a year — and only after you've talked with a dietitian. Then only buy oats made in a gluten-free facility and certified as gluten-free.

FATS For the most part, fats are safe to eat, but you have to be careful. Fats such as olive oil, canola oil, vegetable oils and avocados are all gluten-free. So are nuts and oils made from nuts. Be careful with nut butters, such as peanut butter. Some products may have additives that contain gluten. Look for brands labeled gluten-free or check the ingredients.

Butter and most margarines also are gluten-free, but these products should be used in moderation because they contain saturated fat and trans fats.

It's important to get some fat in your diet because fat is essential to the life and function of your body's cells, and it plays a role in the regulation of many body processes. Most people, however, get far more fat than they need.

Best gluten-free options If you eat a lot of fresh, unprocessed foods, you're already well on your way to getting the best types of fat, while eliminating the types of fat that you don't need. Olive oil, canola oil and vegetable oils are good fat choices. Use these fats when you can. Avocados are another good source of fat.

Be aware that many gluten-free processed foods — foods such as gluten-free chips and gluten-free cookies — may be high in fat. In an effort to enhance the flavor and texture, gluten-free baked goods and other gluten-free processed foods sometimes contain more fat than their regular counterparts made with gluten. Compare labels and look for gluten-free products that don't go overboard on fat.

 SWEETS This food group includes sweeteners, desserts and toppings. Many sweeteners, such as table sugar, are naturally gluten-free. However, the foods they're used in, such as cookies and cakes, are often made with wheat or other sources of gluten. For that reason, you need to be wary of any processed desserts or sweets that aren't specifically labeled as gluten-free.

Also remember that sweets can be high in calories and fat. Be smart about your selections and portion sizes.

Best gluten-free options Naturally gluten-free sweeteners include sugar — powdered, granulated and brown — and sugar substitutes. Honey, maple syrup, corn syrup and molasses also fall into this group. Use these sweeteners for cooking and baking.

Hidden gluten

Some foods that contain gluten are obvious. Others may catch you by surprise. The qualities that gluten brings to bread and baked goods — such as elasticity, chewiness and shape retention — also have value in other products.

And remember, it doesn't have to be a food for gluten to be in it. Here are some unlikely, possible culprits of gluten that you should be aware of:

- Candy
- Communion wafers
- Corn chips
- Dairy substitutes
- Deli and lunch meats
- Energy bars
- Medications (some)
- Modeling clay
- Rice and corn breakfast cereals
- Salad dressings
- Spice blends

If you have celiac disease, these gluten hideouts are noteworthy. If you've gone through all of the effort of changing your meals to eliminate gluten from your diet, you don't want to let a vitamin pill undermine your time and hard work.

Occasionally, medications can be a problem. Wheat starch is used as a binding agent in many different types of prescription and over-the-counter medications. Even worse, there are no requirements for labeling or disclosing gluten used in pills. You may be able to identify some gluten-containing ingredients and starches on a medication label, but there's no way to be sure

When planning your meals, use this plate as a guide to what you should eat and how much. Keep in mind these are general guidelines. Not every meal needs to be structured this way, but if you can imagine all of the food you eat each day served on one big plate, this is approximately how the food groups should be apportioned.

Vegetables and fruits should take up half your plate, with vegetables accounting for more of the mix than fruits. Protein sources should take up about a quarter of the plate. Gluten-free grains should fill the other quarter. Also make sure to add dairy to the mix and include healthy fats.

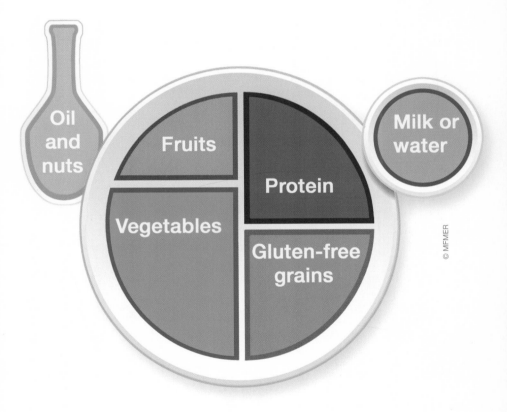

This image can be a regular reminder to keep you on track for eating a balanced diet with all the nutrients that your body needs to heal and stay healthy. Depending on your individual needs, your dietitian may recommend some changes.

whether or not some products are gluten-free just by reading the ingredient list. For more information on medications, see page 194.

Another hidden source of gluten is cross-contamination, which happens when gluten-free foods come into contact with foods that contain gluten. This may happen at your home, in restaurants or at places where food is made.

For example, if you use the same toaster to toast your gluten-free bread as your spouse, who eats regular bread, you're getting gluten by way of cross-contamination. Other kitchen appliances and utensils, such as strainers, cutting boards and measuring spoons, may pose the same problems if they've been used to prepare foods that contain gluten. You'll learn more about how to avoid cross-contamination in Chapter 15.

Putting the pieces together

You now have a general idea about which foods are likely to contain gluten and which aren't. Cheddar cheese is in, but macaroni is out. Jelly is fine, but regular bread is definitely out. Soda is OK but not most beers. Still, you may

Don't forget your vitamins and minerals

In earlier chapters, you learned that celiac disease can affect the body's absorption of important nutrients. It turns out that fixing one problem may produce another. When you steer clear of gluten to help heal your small intestine, you may unintentionally reduce your consumption of important nutrients, including iron and fiber.

Many breakfast cereals, pastas and breads are fortified with vitamins and minerals. When you stop eating these products because they contain gluten, you're missing out on the nutrients these foods contain.

To be clear: You can follow a gluten-free diet and get adequate amounts of key nutrients. Difficulties may arise if you eat only certain foods instead of a variety of foods from the major foods groups. If you have another medical condition, it's also possible you may not get adequate amounts of nutrients.

A dietitian can teach you what foods to eat to replenish nutrients you used to get from foods that are now off-limits. Your doctor or dietitian may also recommend taking a gluten-free multivitamin or supplement.

What about alcohol?

If you're wondering if you can still enjoy an occasional drink of alcohol, the answer is yes, but you need to pick your cocktail carefully.

Distilled liquors — such as brandy, gin, rum, tequila, vodka and whiskey — are all gluten-free. Distilling is a process used in alcohol production that concentrates liquids that have first been brewed. Distilled alcohol doesn't contain any gluten protein, even if the beverage is made with wheat, barley or malt. That's because the gluten protein is too large to survive the distillation process. You have to be careful, though, that gluten-containing flavorings aren't added after production.

Wine is made from fruit and, therefore, is considered gluten-free. However, as with other drinks, be sure to check that additives containing gluten haven't been added. The same is true for wine coolers and hard ciders.

On the flip side, traditional beers, ales, lagers and other malt beverages do contain gluten. These beverages are made from gluten-containing grains and they're not distilled. However, a number of premium and craft brewers have started producing gluten-free beers. Some are brewed with gluten-free grains, such as buckwheat, sorghum, rice and millet. Others are stripped of gluten after processing using special filters and enzymes. So you can still enjoy a frosty mug or pint. Cheers to that!

feel like there are a lot of gaps to fill in, and you're right. In upcoming chapters, you'll gather more details and receive helpful tips on how to read labels, shop and cook gluten-free.

With time, planning and creativity, you'll conquer a brave, new world of delicious gluten-free meals and snacks. Many people find that dinner is the easiest meal to make. That's because many dinner entrees are comprised of different combinations of meat, poultry, fish, potatoes, rice and vegetables — foods you can eat and are easy to prepare.

Gluten-free breakfasts usually aren't much of a stretch either. You may have to give up regular cereal or toast, but there are a number of good gluten-free versions available. Plus, many other common breakfast items are naturally gluten-free, such as eggs and bacon, and cottage cheese and fruit. Most important of all, you don't have to sacrifice your morning coffee!

Snacks are fairly manageable, too. Fruits, vegetables, natural cheeses and nuts are all fair game. You'll find numerous ways to satisfy your hunger when the urge to nibble strikes in between meals.

That leaves lunch and desserts. These tend to be the sticking points for many people. Lunch can be a challenge because it's usually eaten outside the home — at work or at a restaurant — where options are often limited. And, of course, the most commonly packed lunch — the classic sandwich — is a challenge because of the bread. Some people don't find gluten-free bread to be a satisfying substitute for the real deal — it's too dense or too expensive. If you're in this camp, one option is to use a corn tortilla wrap in place of bread. You can also challenge yourself to break out of the sandwich rut and find new ideas for lunch.

If you're a dessert lover, many gluten-free options are delicious by most standards — certainly better than they were a decade ago. The taste of some gluten-free desserts is indistinguishable from the regular versions. Others may not quite live up to the pickiest palates. Take some comfort in knowing that you're not alone in your search for the perfect gluten-free chocolate chip cookie and piecrust. These are subjects of great interest in the gluten-free industry. As more and more manufacturers and bakeries join in the quest for these items, you'll likely benefit from their efforts.

Beyond gluten

If you have celiac disease, you may need to pay attention to food ingredients other than gluten while your small intestine is healing. If gluten has badly damaged your intestine, even some gluten-free foods may cause uncomfortable symptoms such as diarrhea and abdominal pain. This can be a keen source of frustration if you think you're doing everything right in avoiding gluten but you still don't feel right.

LACTOSE INTOLERANCE Lactose is a natural sugar in milk. Some people with celiac disease experience a temporary intolerance to lactose. This intolerance is typically caused by a deficiency of lactase, an enzyme found in the lining of your small intestine. Normally, cells that line the small intestine produce lactase, which breaks lactose in food into smaller sugars that can be absorbed into your bloodstream.

When your small intestine is inflamed, it may not produce enough lactase enzyme. This allows most of the lactose in your food to move undigested into the colon, where intestinal bacteria interact with it. This causes the classic signs and symptoms of lactose intolerance — gas, bloating and diarrhea.

After you stop eating gluten and your small intestine heals, lactose intolerance may go away. Some people, however, develop lactose intolerance independently of celiac disease. In these individuals, the condition may not resolve once celiac disease is under control.

Gluten is commonly found in these foods and beverages. Look for gluten-free versions or avoid them completely:

- Beer
- Breading and coating mixes
- Breads and baked goods, including bagels, cakes, cookies, doughnuts, muffins and pie crusts
- Breakfast foods, including pancakes and waffles
- Candies
- Cereal and granola
- Corn chips
- Crackers, including pretzels and graham crackers
- Croutons
- Deli meats
- Flour and flour tortillas
- French fries
- Gravies
- Imitation meat or seafood, such as mock crab
- Noodles and pastas, including ravioli, dumplings and gnocchi
- Processed lunch meats
- Salad dressings
- Seasoned rice mixes and snack foods, such as potato chips
- Soups and soup bases
- Soy sauce
- Stuffing
- Vegetables in sauce

Don't be surprised if you need to follow a lactose-free diet at the same time as you switch to a gluten-free diet. You'll want to work with a dietitian or your doctor to make sure you're getting enough calcium and vitamin D. Most people with lactose intolerance can tolerate aged cheese, yogurt with active cultures, and small amounts of milk. You might also benefit from lactase-treated milk or taking lactase enzyme supplements when eating dairy products until your body starts producing enough lactase on its own.

Should my whole family go gluten-free?

First of all, remember that celiac disease tends to run in families. If you have celiac disease, it's important that other family members be tested before they eliminate gluten. Eating gluten-free before testing can skew the results.

There's no reason your entire family can't eat gluten-free. A gluten-free diet is a balanced, healthy diet that your whole family can enjoy. Here are some of the pros and cons of making a gluten-free diet a family affair.

During the first few weeks of a gluten-free diet, it can be difficult to know what to eat, and you may worry that you'll eat the wrong thing. Here are some suggestions for easy meals you can make that are gluten-free.

Breakfast
» Gluten-free cereal with banana slices and low-fat milk
» Scrambled eggs with bacon* and a grapefruit half
» Hard-boiled egg, gluten-free bagel and jam, and orange slices
» French toast made with gluten-free bread layered with syrup and peaches
» Gluten-free toast with peanut butter* and orange juice
» Fruit smoothie made with low-fat yogurt* and fresh or frozen fruit
» Vegetable-stuffed omelet with fried potatoes
» Breakfast burrito made of a corn tortilla,* scrambled eggs and salsa

Lunch
» Wraps (tuna salad,* chicken, beef, pork, ham or gluten-free deli meats) on corn tortilla wraps or lettuce wraps with sliced tomatoes and cucumbers
» Chef salad with lettuce, hard-boiled eggs, cheese, ham,* chicken, vegetables and gluten-free salad dressing
» Cheese quesadillas made with corn tortillas,* topped with avocado and salsa
» Cottage cheese* with fresh fruit
» Hot dogs* with baked beans*
» Gluten-free macaroni and cheese (see page 220)
» Peanut butter* on apple slices with a side of yogurt*
» Leftovers from dinner

Dinner
» Roasted chicken and root vegetables, such as carrots, potatoes and onions
» Hamburgers or hot dogs* on gluten-free buns with homemade fries
» Homemade soups or chili
» Chicken tenders with gluten-free breading (see page 222) and fresh fruit salad
» Grilled pork-and-vegetable kebabs over quinoa
» Baked salmon with sour cream* and chives, and steamed green beans
» Stir-fry with vegetables, gluten-free soy sauce and rice
» Gluten-free pizza with a green salad

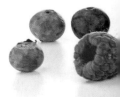

Snacks

* Popcorn — popped in oil (check label if microwaveable or ready-made)
* Fresh fruit
* Ice cream*
* Nuts and raisins
* Gluten-free pretzels
* Gluten-free cereal
* Vegetables with hummus* or gluten-free dip
* String cheese

*Some brands contain gluten. Check the label to be certain.

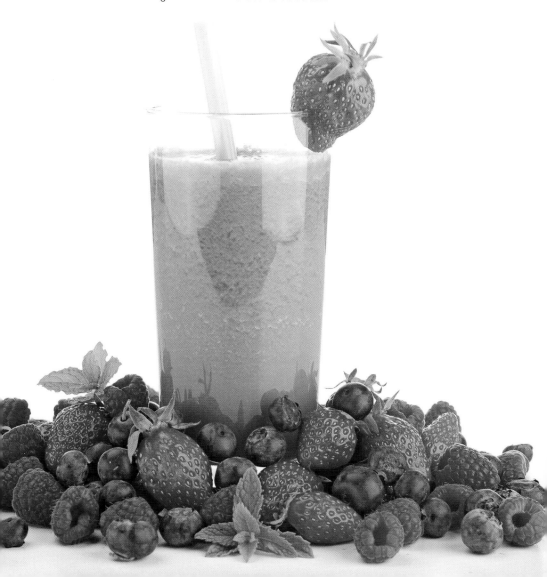

REASONS IN FAVOR For many families, it's hard enough to get one meal on the table every night, in between piano lessons, homework and other commitments, much less two meals — a regular dinner and a gluten-free alternative. It's easy to put more effort into the regular meal for your family than your gluten-free meal. This is no way to fall in love with gluten-free living.

In general, it's easier when the whole family eats gluten-free — at least at home. That way, you're only making one version of every meal. Even better, you don't have to be as concerned about cross-contamination because there are no foods in the house that contain gluten.

Making the transition to a gluten-free diet also is less challenging when the whole family is on board. Face it, it can be downright depressing if the rest of your family is enjoying your favorite pizza and you can't have any. Eventually, you may not mind people eating gluten-filled treats in front of you, but at first it can be more difficult.

If your entire family is eating gluten-free, try to make the endeavor fun. Your family may enjoy sampling new gluten-free recipes. You can even turn the transition into a game with scorecards, blind taste tests, and "gluten-free cookie wars." In the process, your whole family will learn more about healthy eating.

At the very least, it's important to educate your family about gluten-free eating, even if they don't all follow it. If you have kids, they should understand the basic tenets of the diet. Explain the diet to them in terms they can comprehend, based on their ages. Otherwise, the children may be careless about cross-contamination. They may not understand why making a piece of regular toast in the gluten-free toaster is a problem.

REASONS AGAINST There are some drawbacks to having the whole family eat gluten-free. One is cost. Processed gluten-free foods can cost two to five times more than the regular versions. Stocking enough gluten-free foods and beverages for the entire household may boost your grocery bill considerably. Splurging on gluten-free bread, cereal and pasta may not seem like a good investment if some members of the family could easily be eating the regular commercial brands.

Another common obstacle is resentment. Forcing your whole family to give up their favorite foods just because you can't eat them can breed bitterness. For you, there are real health benefits to eating gluten-free. For your family, there aren't. It may not be fair to force them to come along for the ride if there's nothing in it for them. Family members may also become less sympathetic to the challenges you face as you try to eat gluten-free. If you want their support on your gluten-free journey, it's important that their feelings are heard.

Only you know what's best for your family, based on their ages, their eating habits and your household budget. If you want to try an all-for-one-and-one-for-all approach, remember you can always rewrite the rules at any time if it doesn't work. And vice versa. Also, what makes sense for your family may change over time. Be open and willing to come up with your own solutions.

Be prudent, not paranoid

A major change in your diet will take some getting used to. But try not to let the transition overwhelm you and keep you from doing the things you like with the people that you enjoy. Be prudent in your decision-making — sensible, practical and well-advised — but try not to obsess over every detail.

Remember, you can still enjoy family celebrations. You can take your family to a ballgame or a picnic. You can join your co-workers for lunch at a restaurant. You can road-trip to unforgettable destinations. You can do all of these things.

Your long-term goal is to lead a happy and rewarding life that's filled with diverse and satisfying meals. There's a growing community of people who are living gluten-free and genuinely loving it. You're another member of the club.

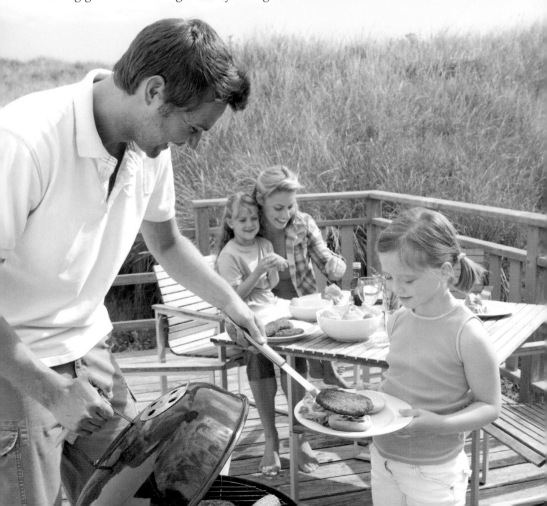

JANELLE'S STORY

My mom was diagnosed with celiac disease just after my daughter was born. Because celiac disease is genetic, she wanted me to be checked. I wasn't having any symptoms, but I tested positive for celiac disease, as did my sister and my dad. Out of a family of four, we're four for four! So far, my two kids have tested negative.

At first, it was completely overwhelming. It seemed like everything I touched had gluten in it. I had a couple of weeks between diagnosis and starting a gluten-free diet. So I had some time to mourn and eat the foods I thought I would never eat again.

Over the last 10 years, it's become so much easier. Now, I can even buy a gluten-free lunch at the school where I work if I want to. And there are a lot of great websites, blogs and resources out there.

At this point, 90 percent of our family meals are gluten-free. My kids are supposed to have some gluten in their diets because they'll be tested for celiac disease throughout their growing-up years. So I buy regular bread for their sandwiches and regular frozen waffles for their breakfasts, but I rarely make two separate meals for dinner.

We eat a lot of fruits and vegetables because they're easy to prepare. We also grill a lot in the summer, and we try a lot of new flavors on the grill. This diet has definitely pushed us to try new things! We eat very few processed foods, and I do a lot of reading before I buy the ones we do eat. Chicken fingers and macaroni and cheese are some of our favorite dinners. I make my chicken fingers with gluten-free breadcrumbs and bake them in the oven. And I make gluten-free macaroni and cheese with real cheese and milk.

When a new gluten-free cookie comes out, we like to sample it, but I don't buy a lot of gluten-free breads and treats. I prefer to make my own. Part of the reason is cost. Why spend $5 for a few gluten-free cookies when I can make a whole batch at home? Plus, I like to know exactly what's going into the cookies. I recently took some homemade cookies to our family and consumer science (FACS) teacher at school, and she said she wouldn't have known they were gluten-free if I hadn't brought them to her. It's good to know that my version is close to the taste of regular cookies. I can't tell because I haven't had the regular ones for so long!

There isn't much I miss on the gluten-free diet now. I can cook almost anything I want, and there are many options for eating out in my hometown. Probably the thing I miss the most is the spontaneity of being able to stop anywhere to eat, especially when we travel.

There's some confusion now that a gluten-free diet has become so popular. Some people view it as a fad. For me it's not — it's necessary for my health.

Glossary of gluten-free grains

As you learn how to eat gluten-free, don't be afraid to experiment. That includes trying different gluten-free whole grains. Whole grains contain important nutrients and fiber, and they're associated with a lower risk of chronic illness, including heart disease, diabetes and cancer. Some of these grains may be unfamiliar to you, but most are prepared in the same way that you would cook regular white rice. Cooking times vary, depending on the consistency of cooked grain you prefer.

Amaranth This ancient grain is high in fiber, iron and protein. It's sold as seeds, puffed or ground into flour. Amaranth is served as a breakfast porridge in many countries. For a modern version, cook amaranth in milk and then stir in cherries, walnuts, maple syrup and cinnamon. You can also pop amaranth seeds like popcorn for a tasty snack.

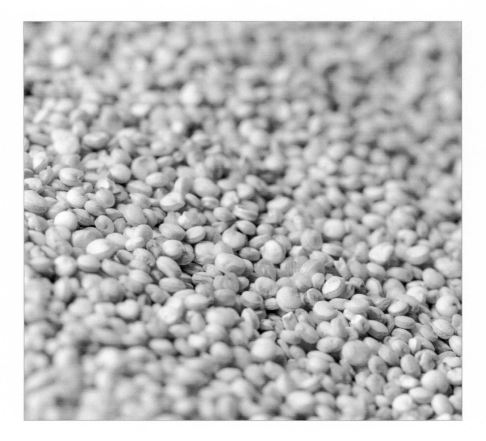

Buckwheat Pure buckwheat is perfect for pancakes and breads. It's also the main ingredient in Japanese soba noodles. Be careful because buckwheat is sometimes mixed with other flours, as in some buckwheat pancake mixes.

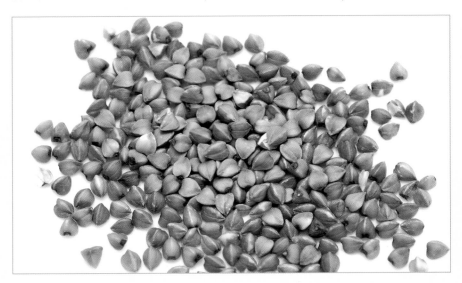

Cornmeal This gluten-free grain is more common than some of the other grains. It's often used in cornbread,* tortillas and muffins, and it's the main ingredient in polenta, a creamy Italian porridge. You can also cool polenta until it's firm and cut it into strips or triangles for baking, grilling or frying. It's crispy without any gluten-containing coating. (*Cornbread often contains wheat flour.)

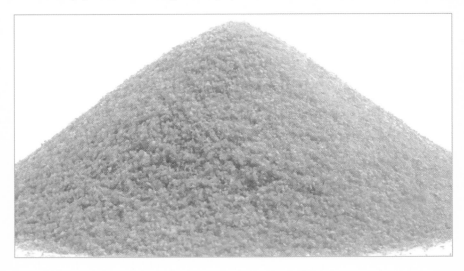

Flax Flaxseeds have a nutty, toasted flavor and lots of nutrients. You can sprinkle them on gluten-free cereal or oatmeal or yogurt with fruit. If you make your own gluten-free granola, flax is a great addition to the recipe. You can also add flaxseeds into homemade gluten-free cookies and granola bars.

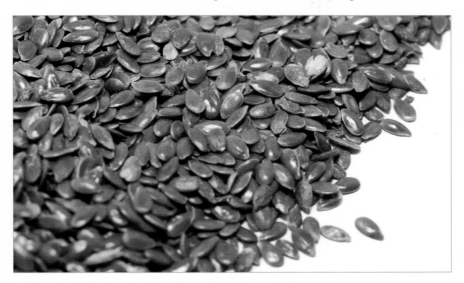

Millet Millet grains are usually small and yellowish. They have a mild flavor that is a nice addition to soups, stews and breads. Millet can also be made into a breakfast cereal.

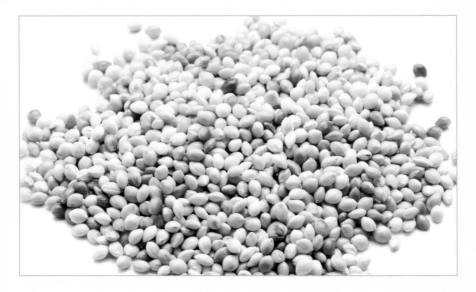

Quinoa This protein-packed superfood is a gluten-free staple. It's light, fluffy, nutty and versatile and cooks in less than 15 minutes. Quinoa (pronounced KEEN-wah) is a quick alternative to pasta or rice, and it can be turned into a savory stuffing. Cooked quinoa is also a great building block for salads. In winter, toss it with dark greens, apples, dried cherries and walnuts. In the summer, mix cooked quinoa with cucumbers, tomatoes, basil or sugar snap peas and your favorite vinaigrette.

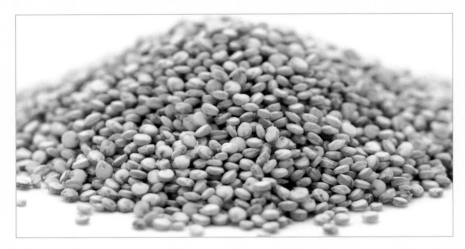

Sorghum This gluten-free grain is about the same size as barley. When toasted, it will puff like tiny popcorn kernels with a sweet, nutty taste. Sorghum can also be substituted for wheat flour in many baked goods.

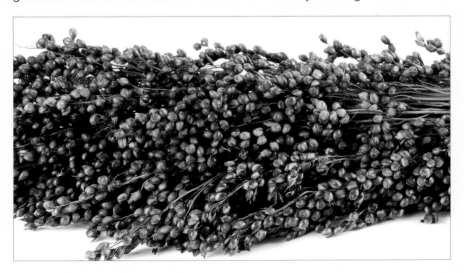

Teff Teff is a tiny Ethiopian grain that's high in iron. It has a sweet, molasses-like flavor that makes for a delicious breakfast cereal. Teff can also be added to baked goods.

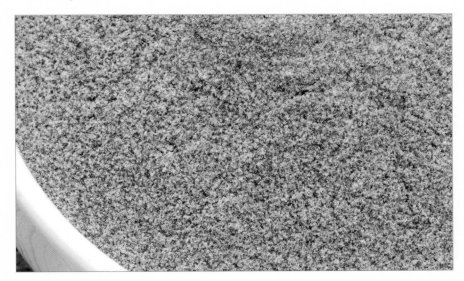

Wild rice Wild rice isn't technically rice. It's the seed of an aquatic grass that's still harvested by Native Americans, mostly in Minnesota. It has a strong flavor so it's often combined with brown rice or white rice or both and sold as a blend. It's delicious in soups and pilafs. It pairs particularly well with chicken and mushrooms.

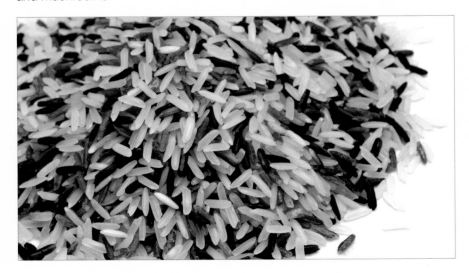

CHAPTER THIRTEEN

Reading food labels

One of the more difficult tasks in eating gluten-free is figuring out what foods contain gluten. There are the obvious sources, such as bread and pasta, but gluten is also found in a lot of foods or ingredients that you might not expect. So, how do you know which products contain gluten? The answer: You're about to become a master at reading food labels!

What you will quickly find out is that gluten is embedded in many common foods. You can find it in baked goods, crackers, cereals and frozen dinners. In addition, wheat and barley often appear as secondary ingredients in a number of products in the form of a breading, coating, thickener or flavor enhancer. In addition, gluten is used in foods as an emulsifier, stabilizer or anti-caking agent.

Many people are surprised by all of the places gluten may be lurking that they didn't expect — in fried chicken, fish sticks, soy sauce, gravy mixes, cheese spreads, salad dressings, pie filling, licorice and many other prepared foods. This is why those first few trips to the grocery store can be time-consuming and frustrating.

Rest assured, though, once you get in the habit of reading food labels and you know what to look for, your grocery shopping trips will become much easier. After a while, you'll have a pretty good idea which foods are safe to eat and which aren't. For some foods, you won't even have to look at the label because you'll know the product contains gluten.

Becoming a master detective

The difficult part is that gluten goes by many different names. When you look at a food label, don't expect to see the word *gluten* spelled out in big, bold letters to let you know that this food is off-limits. Nope. It's not that simple.

An important part of eating gluten-free is learning to decode food labels. In general, reading food labels is a good practice for everyone to follow to help ensure smart food choices and healthy eating. When you're on a gluten-free diet, this skill is absolutely essential.

Careful label reading is your best defense against unwanted or hidden gluten. In addition, understanding the information on a food label will help you compare similar foods and choose what's best for your health. You can use food labels as a tool to eat a nutritious, balanced diet.

A dietitian can be a helpful ally in decoding the language of food labels, but you don't need a dietitian's degree to learn today's label lingo. Food and ingredient labeling has improved dramatically over the years, making it possible to quickly scan labels for the most important information. Because of changes in labeling laws, it's much easier than it once was to determine if a product has gluten in it.

And don't forget that many products that are naturally gluten-free don't have labels — fresh vegetables, fruits, fish, poultry, meat and eggs. You can simply pick these products up and put them in your cart. These are the food staples that should make up the bulk of your grocery cart.

For products that have food labels, get in the habit of reading every single label during every single shopping trip. Manufacturers can change ingredients. That means a brand of crackers that was gluten-free two months ago isn't guaranteed to be gluten-free today. Do a quick check just to be sure, even if you bought the product before. It may take a few extra minutes to verify every box and container, but your health is worth this added effort.

WHAT TO LOOK FOR Food companies are required by law to list some ingredients on their packages in clear terms. Wheat is one of these but gluten isn't. Disclosing the existence of gluten on a food package is completely voluntary.

Fortunately, as the craze for gluten-free foods grows, manufacturers are realizing there's an advantage to declaring the gluten-free status of their ingredients. In addition, gluten-free guidelines have been adopted for the food industry requiring certain criteria be met for a food to be labeled gluten-free.

This is very helpful for shoppers looking for gluten-free products. However, it means that gluten is typically referenced only when it's omitted — and only if the manufacturer wants to do so. Therefore, it can still be difficult to tell

Here's a quick guide to the information that you'll find on a food label.

Servings. Manufacturers must list the serving size in standard measurements — such as cups or pieces. The label also includes servings per container to help you calculate the calories and nutrients in the entire package.

Calories. The calories listed show the amount of calories in one serving. The label also shows how many of these calories come from fat. If you're trying to lose weight in addition to eliminating gluten, use this information to compare the calories in similar products.

Nutrients. At a minimum, the product must list the amounts of total fat, saturated fat, trans fat, cholesterol, sodium, total carbohydrate, fiber, sugar, protein, vitamins A and C, calcium, and iron in one serving. This can help you track if you're getting the nutrients you need in a day — or in the case of fat, cholesterol, sodium and sugar, too much of them.

Percent daily value. This information lets you know how much of certain nutrients you should aim for each day. The percent daily value is based on a 2,000- or 2,500-calorie-a-day diet.

Ingredients. All of the ingredients in the product are listed here. This is where you'll find out if the food contains gluten. Food allergy statements also are here.

Nutrition Facts

Serving Size 1 cup (28 g)
Children Under 4 - ¾ cup (21g)
Servings Per Container About 14
Children Under 4 - about 19

Amount Per Serving	Cereal	with ½ cup skim milk	Cereal for Children under 4
Calories	100	150	80
Calories from Fat	15	20	10
		% Daily Value**	
Total Fat 2g*	3%	3%	1.5g
Saturated Fat 0.5g	3%	3%	1.5g
Trans Fat			0g
Polyunsaturated Fat 0.5g			0.5g
Monounsaturated Fat 1.5g			0.5g
Cholesterol 0mg	0%	1%	0mg
Sodium 140mg	6%	8%	105mg
Potassium 180mg	5%	11%	135mg
Total Carbohydrate 20g	7%	9%	15g
Dietary Fiber 3g	11%	11%	2g
Soluble Fiber 1g			0g
Sugars 1g			1g
Other carbohydrate 16g			16g
Protein 3g			2g

		% Daily Value**	
Protein*	-	-	9%
Vitamin A	10%	15%	10%
Vitamin C	10%	10%	10%
Calcium	10%	25%	8%
Iron	45%	45%	50%
Vitamin D	10%	25%	6%
Thiamin	25%	30%	35%
Riboflavin	2%	10%	2%
Niacin	25%	25%	35%
Vitamin B₆	25%	25%	45%
Folic Acid	50%	50%	60%
Vitamin B₁₂	25%	30%	30%
Phosphorus	10%	20%	8%
Magnesium	8%	10%	10%
Zinc	25%	30%	30%

* Amount in cereal. A serving of cereal plus skim milk provides 2g total fat, less than 5mg cholesterol, 200mg sodium, 380mg potassium, 26g total carbohydrate (7g sugars0, and 8g protein.)
** Percent Daily Values are based on a 2,000 calorie diet. Your daily values may be higher or lower depending on your calorie needs:

	Calories	2,000	2,500
Total Fat	Less than	65g	80g
Sat. Fat	Less than	20g	25g
Cholesterol	Less than	300mg	300mg
Sodium	Less than	2,400mg	2,400mg
Potassium		3,500mg	3,500mg
Total Carbohydrate		300g	375g
Dietary Fiber		25g	30g
Protein		50g	65g

Ingredients: Whole Grain Oats, Corn Starch, Sugar, Salt, Tripotassium Phosphate, Wheat Starch, Vitamin E (mixed tocopherols). **Added to Preserve Freshness.**

Vitamins and Minerals: Calcium Carbonate, Iron and Zinc (mineral nutrients), **Vitamin C** (sodium ascorbate), **A B Vitamin** (niacinamide), **Vitamin B₆** (pyridoxine hydrochloride), **Vitamin A** (palmitate), **Vitamin B1** (thaimin monotrate), **A B Vitamin** (folic acid), **Vitaimin B₁₂, Vitamin D₃.**

© MFMER

when a product does contain gluten. Your best bet is to follow this simple five-step approach:

1. Look for a gluten-free logo or claim on the package.
2. Check the list of ingredients for evidence of wheat.
3. Look for barley (including malt), rye and oats in the ingredient list.
4. Be alert to any risk of cross-contamination.
5. Contact the product manufacturer if needed.

Step 1: Look for a gluten-free logo or claim

Gluten-free foods may be labeled with a variety of different logos or phrases that can appear anywhere on the package. You're looking for the following statements:

⇢ "Gluten-free"
⇢ "No gluten"
⇢ "Free of gluten"
⇢ "Without gluten"

Gluten-free labeling is voluntary. If a product includes such a statement, it falls under the gluten-free food label ruling recently issued by the Food and Drug Administration (FDA). This regulation standardizes what "gluten-free" means on a food label. If you're holding a product containing such a logo or phrase, that product must contain less than 20 parts per million (ppm) of gluten — an amount considered by health experts to be gluten-free.

This regulation applies to all foods regulated by the FDA sold in the United States, including those imported from other countries. Companies who choose to use this label are accountable to the FDA.

Before the FDA ruling, there was no legal definition or national standard for the food industry to use in labeling products as gluten-free. As a result, various manufacturers and certifying organizations developed their own thresholds for gluten-free claims. This created significant confusion. It was nearly impossible for even the most careful shopper to know how much gluten was in a product labeled gluten-free.

Not surprisingly, an increasing number of manufacturers are now going out of their way to label products that meet the criteria as gluten-free. They know this label can translate into big profits.

WHAT IT MEANS The FDA ruling doesn't require manufacturers to test their products to make sure they meet all requirements. However, manufacturers will face charges from the FDA if they don't comply with the standards and the product may be removed from the market. The FDA can monitor products through review of food labels, on-site inspections and food sample analysis. So it's in a manufacturer's best interests to verify that their products are well within the limits.

Even foods that are naturally gluten-free can be stamped with a gluten-free label. That's why you may see gluten-free logos or claims on items such as bottled spring water, fresh salmon and fresh berries. The label guarantees that the product doesn't contain any gluten-containing grains or ingredients derived from gluten-containing grains, and it guarantees the product wasn't manufactured in a facility where it may have become contaminated during processing. Any potential cross-contamination of gluten during processing is factored into the 20 ppm limit.

Don't assume that if the product doesn't contain a gluten-free claim or logo that it contains gluten. Remember that gluten-free labeling is optional. Foods without a label may be gluten-free and safe — or they may not.

CERTIFICATION LOGOS You may notice some products contain gluten-free certification logos. These logos indicate that the product has been tested to ensure it doesn't contain gluten. There are several independent gluten-free certification programs in the United States — including those backed by the Celiac Sprue Association, the Gluten-Free Certification Organization and the National Foundation for Celiac Awareness.

Each certification program has its own symbol and its own requirements for certification. However, all are safely within the boundary set by the FDA — usually less than 10 or even 5 ppm of gluten. The FDA doesn't endorse or recommend any of these certification programs, but it does allow food companies to use the logos, as long as they're not misleading or untruthful. The emblems are a visible cue that the product meets FDA regulations and contains under 20 ppm of gluten — often less.

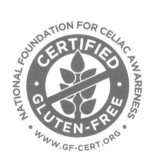 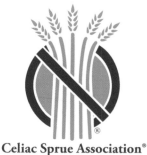 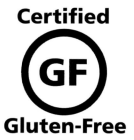

© National Foundation for Celiac Awareness, Celiac Sprue Association and Gluten Intolerance Group. Used with permission.

These logos indicate the product has been tested to ensure it meets FDA requirements.

Different agencies, different rules

The Food and Drug Administration's gluten-free labeling regulations apply to all foods and beverages that are under the jurisdiction of the FDA. In general, most products that you see at the grocery store are covered under this ruling. This includes packaged foods, canned foods, frozen foods and dairy products.

There are some foods and beverages, however, that fall outside of the FDA's reach. Meat, poultry and egg products are regulated by the United States Department of Agriculture (USDA). They don't have to adhere to FDA gluten-free labeling guidelines. Alcoholic beverages — including distilled spirits, wines with 7 percent or more alcohol, and malt beverages made with barley and hops — are regulated by the Alcohol and Tobacco Tax and Trade Bureau (TTB). They're also exempt from FDA regulations.

These government organizations handle gluten-free labeling and allergen labeling a little differently. Both the USDA and the TTB encourage manufacturers to list allergens — such as wheat — on their product labels. However, allergen listings aren't mandatory like they are on products under the jurisdiction of the FDA. Fortunately, many manufacturers comply anyway, so check the label.

To date, the USDA hasn't adopted any rules related to gluten-free labeling. The TTB has an interim policy that states a gluten-free label may be placed on alcoholic beverages made from ingredients that don't contain gluten and that meet the FDA definition of gluten-free.

In other words, a gluten-free label is only allowed on beverages that are naturally gluten-free, such as wines and certain distilled alcohols. You may also see gluten-free claims or logos on specialized beers made with sorghum, rice or wheat — instead of the traditional malted barley or hops. These specialized beers don't meet the definition for "beer" established by the TTB. As a result, the FDA oversees the gluten-free brews. They can sport a gluten-free label if they have less than 20 parts per million (ppm) of gluten, as defined in the FDA ruling.

Beer made from traditional barley or hops that have been specially processed to remove the gluten must use one of the following statements. The beverages must also include a qualifying statement that the product may contain gluten:
+ "Processed to remove gluten"
+ "Treated to remove gluten"
+ "Crafted to remove gluten"

Manufacturers of vitamins and minerals also are not regulated by the FDA. If a supplement claims to be gluten-free, that doesn't mean it meets gluten-free labeling regulations. For more on medications, see page 194.

Don't assume too much Remember that just because a product is labeled gluten-free doesn't mean it's healthy. Some gluten-free products contain a lot of fat, sugar or food additives. That's why you also want to look at the food nutrition label to see what's in the food.

In addition, don't assume that because a certain manufacturer has some gluten-free foods that all of the products it markets are made without gluten. Labels and logos apply to individual food products, not a whole food line. If you find a particular gluten-free brand or manufacturer you like, make sure to look for a gluten-free label on every product every time. As mentioned earlier, manufacturing processes change. Just because that particular food item is gluten-free today doesn't mean it will be forever.

Why gluten-free isn't completely 'free'

You might be a bit troubled by the fact that a "gluten-free" product can actually contain some gluten. Shouldn't a gluten-free label mean that a product has zero gluten?

The Food and Drug Administration (FDA) selected a maximum limit of less than 20 parts per million (ppm) for foods that carry the gluten-free label for a few reasons. For one, 20 ppm is the lowest level that can reliably and consistently be detected in a variety of food forms. Second, this limit is in line with the criteria used in some other countries. And finally, because foods can be contaminated with trace amounts of gluten during the food manufacturing and handling process, a zero-tolerance policy outside of a lab environment is nearly impossible. A level below 20 ppm would make it far more difficult for manufacturers to offer gluten-free products.

In addition, removing absolutely all gluten is unnecessary. Most people with celiac disease can tolerate very small amounts of gluten. Although it's difficult to pinpoint an exact number, scientists and doctors generally agree that 20 ppm is safe for most people. How much is 20 ppm? The proportion is the same as .002 percent. That's not very much.

Keep in mind that many products labeled as gluten-free are well under the 20 ppm cap. And a lot of the foods you eat each day, such as fruit, vegetables and meat, are naturally and genuinely gluten-free.

Step 2: Seek out wheat

If a product doesn't have a gluten-free label, your next step is to look for indications that the product is made with wheat. To be clear, "wheat-free" isn't the same as "gluten-free." So your search can't end with wheat.

However, wheat is a major source of gluten in food products in the United States, so it's the logical next step after looking for a gluten-free label. Wheat can appear in many forms under many names. To see if a product contains wheat, look for these terms on the ingredients list:

- Dextrin
- Dinkle
- Durum
- Einkorn
- Emmer
- Farina
- Graham flour
- Kamut
- Semolina
- Spelt
- Wheat berry
- Wheat germ
- Wheat gluten
- Wheat bran
- Wheat starch

Luckily, you don't have to weed through all of this jargon, thanks to the FDA Food Allergen Labeling and Consumer Protection Act (FALCPA). According to this act, food manufacturers are legally required to list the eight most common foods that trigger food allergies (food allergens). Most other countries have similar rules. In the United States, information about food allergies has to be written in simple terms that adults and older children can understand. The eight common foods that trigger food allergies are: milk, eggs, peanuts, tree nuts, fish, shellfish, soy and wheat.

Labels must list the type of food allergen, as well as any ingredient that contains a protein from the eight major food allergens. This includes any allergens found in flavorings, colorings or other additives.

Essentially, if a food product contains any type of wheat or a derivative of wheat, such as flour or starch, it will be clearly identified. Food manufacturers are required to identify the wheat in one of two ways. They can include an allergy statement after the ingredient list, which typically starts with the word "contains," as shown in Figure 1 on page 190. Otherwise, the food allergen can be listed in the ingredient list, as shown in Figure 2.

Figure 1

Nutrition Facts

Serving Size 1 oz. (28 g/ About 17 pretzels)
Servings Per Container About 16

Amount Per Serving		
Calories	110	
Calories from Fat	10	
		% Daily Value**
Total Fat 1g*		**2%**
Saturated Fat 0g		**0%**
Trans Fat 0g		
Cholesterol 0mg		**0%**
Sodium 450mg		**19%**
Potassium 80mg		**2%**
Total Carbohydrate 23g		**8%**
Dietary Fiber 1g		**4%**
Sugars less than 1g		
Protein 2g		
		% Daily Value**
Vitamin A		0%
Vitamin C		0%
Calcium		0%
Iron		6%
Thiamin		8%
Riboflavin		8%
Niacin		6%
Phosphorus		2%
Magnesium		2%

* Percent Daily Values are based on a 2,000 calorie diet. Your daily values may be higher or lower depending on your calorie needs:

	Calories	2,000	2,500
Total Fat	Less than	65g	80g
Sat. Fat	Less than	20g	25g
Cholesterol	Less than	300mg	300mg
Sodium	Less than	2,400mg	2,400mg
Potassium		3,500 mg	3,500mg
Total Carbohydrate		300g	375g
Dietary Fiber		25g	30g

Calories per gram:
Fat   9
Carbohydrate 4
Protein   4

Ingredients: Enriched Flour (wheat flour, niacin, reduced iron, thiamin mononitrate, riboflavin, folic acid), Salt, Corn Oil, Corn Syrup, Ammonium Bicarbonate, Malt Extract, and Yeast.

Contains Wheat Ingredient.

No Preservatives.

Ingredients: **Enriched Flour** (wheat flour, niacin, reduced iron, thiamin mononitrate, riboflavin, folic acid), **Salt, Corn Oil, Corn Syrup, Ammonium Bicarbonate, Malt Extract, and Yeast.**

Contains Wheat Ingredient.

No Preservatives.

Figure 2

Nutrition Facts

Serving Size 1 oz. (28 g/ About 12 chips)
Servings Per Container About 9

Amount Per Serving		
Calories	150	
Calories from Fat	70	
		% Daily Value**
Total Fat 8g*		**12%**
Saturated Fat 1g		**5%**
Trans Fat 0g		
Polyunsaturated Fat 2.5g		
Monounsaturated Fat 4g		
Cholesterol 0mg		**0%**
Sodium 140mg		**12%**
Potassium 180mg		**2%**
Total Carbohydrate 16g		**5%**
Dietary Fiber 3g		**4%**
Sugars 1g		
Protein 2g		
		% Daily Value**
Vitamin A		0%
Vitamin C		2%
Calcium		2%
Iron		2%
Thiamin		2%
Riboflavin		4%
Phosphorus		8%
Magnesium		6%

* Percent Daily Values are based on a 2,000 calorie diet. Your daily values may be higher or lower depending on your calorie needs:

	Calories	2,000	2,500
Total Fat	Less than	65g	80g
Sat. Fat	Less than	20g	25g
Cholesterol	Less than	300mg	300mg
Sodium	Less than	2,400 mg	2,400mg
Potassium		3,500 mg	3,500mg
Total Carbohydrate		300g	375g
Dietary Fiber		25g	30g

Calories per gram:
Fat   9
Carbohydrate 4
Protein   4

Ingredients: Ground Yellow Corn, Corn, Sunflower Oil and/or Canola Oil, Salt, Whey (milk), Dry Buttermilk. Romano Cheese (cultured pasteurized part-skim, salt and enzymes.) Tomato Powder, Cheddar Cheese (cultured pasteurized part-skim, salt and enzymes), Onion Powder, Partially Hydrogenated Soybean Oil, Disodium Phosphate, Garlic Powder, Wheat Flour, Natural and Artificial Flavor, Parmesan Cheese (cultured pasteurized part-skim, salt and enzymes), Dextrose, Lactic Acid, Spice, Artificial Color (yellow 6, extractives of turmeric and caramel color), Disodium Inosinate, and not more than 2% Silicon Dioxide added as an anti-caking agent. (May contain Soy Beans).

© MFMER

enzymes.) **Tomato Powder, Cheddar Cheese** (cultured pasteurized part-skim, salt and enzymes), **Onion Powder, Partially Hydrogenated Soybean Oil, Disodium Phosphate, Garlic Powder, Wheat Flour, Natural and Artificial Flavor, Parmesan Cheese** (cultured pasteurized part-skim, salt and enzymes), **Dextrose, Lactic Acid, Spice, Artificial Color** (yellow 6, extractives of turmeric and

If you have a wheat allergy or you need to avoid gluten, steer clear if you see wheat listed on a food label in either of these ways. If it contains wheat, it contains gluten.

Step 3: Search for barley, rye and oats

These gluten-containing ingredients are much more difficult to identify than wheat, because they're not considered allergens. They don't have to be listed in plain language or in an allergy statement, and they can appear in some unexpected places. So you'll need to learn some code names for these sources of gluten.

BARLEY OR MALT Barley may be used as a thickener in soups and stews. It's also commonly used to enhance flavor. Products made from barley may include the words *barley* or *malt*, the most common form of barley. Be on the lookout for any products that contain:

- Barley extract
- Barley flavoring
- Malt
- Malt flavoring
- Malt extract
- Malt sugar
- Malt vinegar

Barley and malt are commonly used in cereals, malted milk, beer, rice milk, rice syrups, protein bars and snack foods.

Contrary to how it appears, maltodextrin is OK to eat. It's made from corn. Also, maltose is technically a sugar made from barley, but it's typically refined, in which the protein is removed, making it gluten-free.

RYE Of course, rye is found in rye bread, but it may also be in other bakery items, including other bread products and crackers. Rye is also crossbred with wheat to create triticale. However, companies are required to list triticale as a wheat allergen.

OATS In general, it's a good idea to avoid oats in various forms — rolled oats, steel-cut oats, oatmeal and oat berries — unless you know they're gluten-free. Watch for oats in baked goods, snack foods, cereals and granola bars, unless the products are labeled gluten-free. Oats are also used as a thickening ingredient in some prepared foods.

Step 4: Look for cross-contamination warnings

Cross-contamination can occur when gluten-free products inadvertently mingle with those containing gluten during milling, shipping and manufacturing. As a result, the gluten-free products become tainted.

If you have celiac disease, gluten from cross-contamination can be danger-ous. If a product has a gluten-free label, it's a promise that any gluten from cross-contamination is below the required threshold. However, in the absence of a gluten-free label, you may need to do some detective work to determine if a product might contain gluten from manufacturing processes.

Food labeling laws require food allergens to be identified even in very small amounts — but only when they're contained as an ingredient. Manufacturers aren't required to include warnings about food allergens accidentally intro-duced during manufacturing or packaging.

Cross-contamination may occur more commonly than you think. One small study tested 22 samples of naturally gluten-free grains, seeds and flours to see how much cross-contamination existed. More than 30 percent were found to have gluten levels greater than 20 ppm.

WARNINGS The good news is that many manufacturers voluntarily include warnings about cross-contamination, even though they're not required to do so. These advisory labels, which appear below the ingredient list, aren't always prominent, however, so you have to look for them. And, manufactur-ers have different ways of saying that cross-contamination may be present. For example, labels may say, "Manufactured in a factory that also processes wheat," or "Made on shared equipment." The FDA is working to make the format of these advisory labels more consistent so that it's easier to identify products that may contain allergens from cross-contamination.

In the meantime, pay attention to any warnings that you do see. If there's any mention that the product may be contaminated with wheat, it's best to pass on it.

Unfortunately, you won't find cross-contamination warnings related to barley, rye or oats. Similar to allergy statements, manufacturers only post cross-contamination warnings about the eight ingredients that most com-monly cause allergies. This covers wheat, but not other gluten-containing grains.

Step 5: Contact the manufacturer

If a food product is marked with a gluten-free label, it's a clear sign that the product is gluten-free according to the FDA definition. You can safely put products with this label into your grocery cart and head for the checkout.

If a food doesn't contain such a label, you need to put your detective skills to work to determine if it does or doesn't contain gluten. Despite your best efforts at an exhaustive search for gluten, you may worry that you missed something. Or you may have questions about the terms that you're seeing on a label.

As you attempt to sort out which foods do and don't contain gluten, you may find it helpful to purchase a gluten-free shopping guide. These guides provide a thorough, confirmed list of tens of thousands of gluten-free foods and beverages. They cover major name brands, as well as store brands from the most common grocery store chains. They can be very helpful when you make the switch to a gluten-free diet and you're not yet an expert at interpreting food labels.

Most guides are compact, so you can easily take them to the grocery store and refer to them as you select canned soups, cereals, ice cream and other products. You can also use them to find specific brands that you can order online. Plus, you may be relieved to see how extensive the guides are. (There are hundreds of pages of things that you can eat!) A dietitian can help you find a reliable shopping guide.

Just beware that shopping guides aren't a replacement for label reading and savvy shopping. Manufacturers can change product ingredients at any time. So even if the guides are 100 percent accurate the day they're sent to the printer, they could contain some false information by the time you receive them. Use the guide as a shortcut to help you narrow down your choices, but make sure to double-check the ingredient list before you put the product in your grocery cart.

Also make sure you're always using the latest edition of any shopping guide. Many guides are published annually. Buy a new version whenever it's available so that your list is always as current as possible. Some guides are also affiliated with websites that post updates as products change.

Another way to access product information is with a mobile app. Some apps contain a huge database of gluten-free items available at grocery stores, restaurants and fast-food chains. Plus, they're updated regularly, so you always have the latest gluten infor-mation. Other apps contain general tips and advice on label reading, dining at various ethnic restaurants and living gluten-free. Take advantage of technology tools that you find handy and helpful.

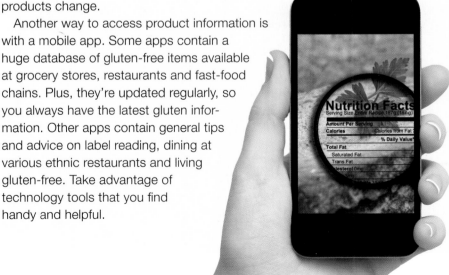

If you have any doubt about whether a product contains gluten after reading the label, contact the manufacturer. You can usually find a phone number located on the food label. Otherwise, look up the product or manufacturer on the Internet.

When you call a food manufacturer, generally you'll reach a consumer information department. Inquire about the specific information that you need. Be as precise and concise as possible about your personal dietary needs.

You may also be able to email the manufacturer or submit a request for information on the company's website. Many manufacturers include detailed nutrient and ingredient information on their websites. Information about gluten is sometimes included in the frequently asked questions (FAQ) section.

Because interest in gluten is increasing, more manufacturers are regularly receiving questions about it, and they may have answers at the ready. If the manufacturer can't answer your questions to your satisfaction, consider spending your money with manufacturers that can.

Medication and supplement labels

Gluten isn't only found in foods. It's hidden in all sorts of unlikely places, including medications and multivitamins. The adhesive substances that bind together the contents of pills or tablets, called excipients, may contain gluten.

An excipient is an inactive ingredient, meaning it doesn't have any therapeutic effect. But just because it's inactive doesn't mean it's harmless. Dyes, preservatives and flavoring agents found in medications and supplements can cause allergic reactions in some individuals. Among people with celiac disease, gluten can damage the small intestine.

It's important to read the labels of any supplements and over-the-counter medications you purchase. In addition, make sure to let your pharmacist know you can't take prescription medications that contain gluten. Be aware that inactive ingredients in comparable brand and generic medications aren't always the same. If you switch from a brand medication to a generic drug or from one generic pill to another brand, you'll need to recheck the inactive ingredients to be sure you're not getting any gluten.

MEDICATIONS Unfortunately, prescription and over-the-counter medications don't fall under the gluten-free labeling rule. There are no requirements for labeling gluten or other common allergens found in medications. However, you can look for signs of gluten in the list of inactive ingredients on the Drug Facts label (see the opposite page).

The following ingredients may be associated with gluten. Avoid packages with these terms or investigate them further:

Drug Facts

Active ingredients (in each tablet)	Purpose
Cholorpheniramine maleate 2 mg	Antihistamine

Uses temporarily relieves these symptoms due to hay fever or other upper respiratory allergies:
■ sneezing ■ runny nose ■ itchy, watery eyes ■ itchy throat

| Cholorpheniramine maleate 2 mg | Antihistamine |

Warnings
Ask a doctor before you use if you have
■ glaucoma ■ a breathing problem such as emphysema or chronic bronchitis
■ trouble urinating due to enlarged prostate gland

Ask a doctor or pharmacist before use if you are taking tranquilizers or sedatives

When using this product
■ drowsiness may occur ■ avoid alcoholic drinks
■ alcohol, sedatives, and tranquilizers may increase drowsiness
■ be careful when driving a motor vehicle or operating machinery
■ excitability may occur, especially in children

If pregnant or breast-feeding, ask a health professional before use.
Keep out of reach of children. In case of overdose, get medical help or contact a Poison Control Center right away.

Directions

adults and children 12 years and over	take 2 tablets every 4 to 6 hours; not more than 12 tablets in 24 hours
children 6 years to under 12 years	take 1 tablet every 4 to 6 hours; not more than 6 tablets in 24 hours
children under 6 years	ask a doctor

© MFMER

Drug Facts (continued)

Other information ■ store at 20-25 C (68-77 F) ■ protect from excessive moisture
Inactive ingredients D&C yellow no.10, lactose magnesium stearate, microcrystalline cellulose, pregelatinized starch

Inactive ingredients D&C yellow cellulose, pregelatinized starch

↔ Wheat or wheat starch

↔ Modified starch (not specified as corn or another gluten-free source)

↔ Pregelatinized starch (not specified as corn or another gluten-free source)

↔ Pregelatinized modified starch (not specified as corn or another gluten-free source)

↔ Maltodextrin (not specified as corn or another gluten-free source)

↔ Dextri-maltose (which may contain barley malt)

↔ Caramel coloring (which may contain barley malt)

↔ Dextrin (usually comes from corn or potato, but worth checking)

Because the sources of the inactive ingredients aren't always listed, you may need to call the manufacturer to determine if a product is gluten-free.

DIETARY SUPPLEMENTS Unlike medications, dietary supplements, including vitamins, are regulated by the Food and Drug Administration (FDA). They must comply with the Food Allergen Labeling and Consumer Protection Act (FALCPA), which requires manufacturers to clearly list common allergens on their packages, including wheat. The products also fall under the August 2013 gluten-free food labeling rule. If a vitamin or supplement is labeled as gluten-free, it must contain less than 20 parts per million (ppm) of gluten.

All of this means that you can check a dietary supplement bottle for gluten in the same way that you would check a bottle of barbecue sauce for gluten. Look for a gluten-free label, but remember that gluten-free labeling is voluntary. Next, check the Supplement Facts label for signs of wheat allergens. This helps you quickly rule out any products that contain wheat, although wheat isn't the only source of gluten. Finally, scrutinize the list of ingredients for possible gluten. If you can't tell for sure, call the manufacturer.

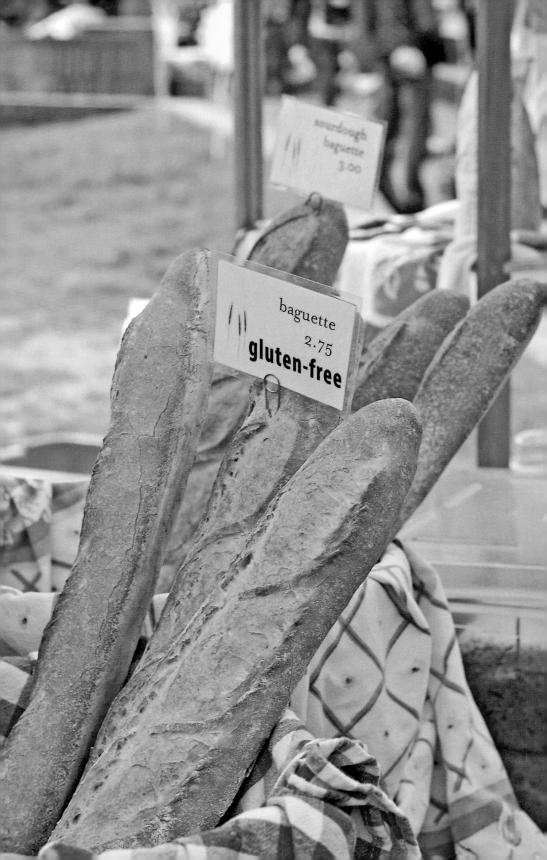

sourdough
baguette
3.00

baguette
2.75
gluten-free

THE BOTTOM LINE Don't forgo a recommended medication or supplement because it's difficult to tell if a product is gluten-free. But also don't take any chances. Work with your pharmacist to be certain the product is safe and if you need to, find alternatives. It's also a good idea to periodically recheck the pills that you're taking, because manufacturers can change the source of inactive ingredients.

Be vigilant

The 2013 gluten-free food labeling ruling goes a long way toward protecting consumers against false claims and deceptive advertising surrounding gluten-free foods. With this ruling in place, food manufacturers who don't live up to their gluten-free labels can face the FDA charge of misbranding.

You can be certain that manufacturers of gluten-free foods are under a great deal of scrutiny from the FDA. They're also feeling the heat from a large community of people who have celiac disease and related disorders who aren't afraid to report products that contain too much gluten. However, this ruling doesn't necessarily mean that every independent baker, deli and coffee shop is adhering to the FDA law.

If you find a loaf of bread that's labeled "gluten-free" at your local farmer's market or bakery and it seems unlike any other gluten-free loaf you've ever seen, ask lots of questions. Venders can make honest mistakes. Sometimes products get mixed up in the course of a busy day, so they aren't labeled properly. Sometimes venders don't fully understand all of the foods and ingredients that contain gluten, and they mistakenly apply a "gluten-free" label to a product that really isn't. Sometimes venders aren't educated on cross-contamination. Sometimes people assume that if it's free of wheat, it's gluten-free. And, of course, there is a small group of unscrupulous sellers who know their products aren't really gluten-free, but they use the label anyway.

Trust your instincts about what you're seeing and tasting. If you bought food that was labeled gluten-free, but you have a sense that something's wrong, stop and ask questions. Don't keep eating something that you think might contain gluten.

Also beware that the FDA ruling doesn't stop manufacturers and celebrities from claiming — or implying — that a gluten-free diet is healthier or will help you lose weight. Be cautious about buying gluten-free products that promise weight loss, increased energy and other health benefits. While these products may be gluten-free, they may not live up to all of their claims.

In the next chapter, we'll talk about what foods to purchase on your next grocery shopping trip to ensure you have the right supply of gluten-free foods in your kitchen for cooking and eating.

CHAPTER FOURTEEN

Restocking your kitchen

Whether your kitchen is the heart of your home or the place where you store the basics — food and the microwave — it needs to become gluten-safe, just like your diet. When you first adopt a gluten-free diet, your goal is to focus on eating simple foods that are naturally gluten-free. Often, the easiest way to do this is to make your meals yourself. To do that, you need to make sure your kitchen is supplied with the right foods and set up properly.

If you don't consider yourself a cook and you're not comfortable in the kitchen, don't worry. You don't need to be a professional chef to make delicious gluten-free meals. Creating tasty gluten-free meals can be as simple as assembling gluten-free ingredients.

You can make quick bean burritos by microwaving black beans and cheese and wrapping them in corn tortillas with avocado, salsa or sour cream. You can scramble eggs along with your favorite vegetables. You can top prewashed salad greens with canned tuna, tomatoes, cucumbers, lemon and olive oil. Or, you can just smear a crisp ripe apple with gluten-free peanut butter.

It all starts by making sure your kitchen has been cleaned so that it doesn't contain any gluten remnants. To eat gluten-free, you need a safe workspace. Next, you'll want to fill that workspace with healthy ingredients. This chapter will help you de-gluten and restock your kitchen — from the refrigerator to the countertops and cabinets. Once you have the right foods and cooking gear on hand, you can create gluten-free meals and snacks with ease.

How to begin

Once you learn that you need to avoid gluten, your natural inclination may be to stage a quick coup. Many people feel they need to immediately head for the pantry, toss everything in there and replace it all with gluten-free versions.

Not everything in your pantry will need to go because not everything contains gluten. The best approach is to carefully examine what you have on hand, do a thorough cleaning, and restock your kitchen with the right foods.

INVENTORY YOUR PANTRY AND FRIDGE Many foods that you may already love are naturally gluten-free. These include fresh fruits and vegetables (and plain canned or frozen versions), as well as rice, beans, nuts, fresh meat, poultry and fish, milk, eggs, cheese, corn tortillas, plain pickles, plain chocolate, and jelly. However, if you haven't been on the lookout for gluten until now, you may have inadvertently purchased some of these foods with added ingredients that do contain gluten. So you need to look at each label.

Take a morning or an afternoon to inventory all of the foods that you currently have in your home. This will take at least a few hours. Turn on some good music. Pour yourself something to drink. And settle into this project.

Start by emptying all of the food out of your pantry, cupboards, refrigerator and spice racks. You can use a cooler for refrigerated or frozen foods, if you need to. You might start with one big pile on the floor or countertops, but your goal is to separate the items into two piles:
  → Definitely gluten-free
  → Definitely not gluten-free, or not sure

This will be a big test of your newfound label-reading skills. You'll need to check every bottle, can, jar, bag and seasoning packet. If the products are old or labels are missing or difficult to read, place them in the "not sure" pile. Don't take any chances. Expect that your kitchen may look like a disaster in the process. That's OK.

Also remember that any food items that were manufactured before the August 2013 gluten-free labeling laws went into full effect may not meet the new standards. If you have older items that are labeled gluten-free, you aren't guaranteed that they contain less than 20 parts per million of gluten. You'll need to look for other clues to determine if the product contains gluten.

You can also take this opportunity to chuck out any cans that are badly dented, bulging, rusty or leaky or that have broken seals. Even if their contents are completely gluten-free, you don't want them. They could be spoiled. The same holds true for foods that are out of date.

Finally, assume that all opened spreads — such as peanut butter, butter, cream cheese, mayonnaise, mustard, jelly, jam and chutney — are probably contaminated with gluten. The same is true of opened baking ingredients, such as sugar, baking soda and baking powder. Someone may have inadvertently double-dipped a knife or measuring spoon that has touched regular bread or flour into these products. Most people do this routinely — until they learn that they have to avoid gluten. Put all of these products in your "not sure" pile.

Write down your 'must haves'

After sorting through the food in your kitchen, look at the definitely not gluten-free and not sure pile. Chances are it contains a lot of items like soup, dry pasta, chips, crackers, salad dressings and other items. Jot down the items you use frequently that are in this pile. These are the items you'll want to reach for when you prepare a meal or are hungry for a snack.

To help you ease into your new diet, look for gluten-free replacements for these foods. These items can be the beginning of your shopping list. You'll be surprised how many gluten-free substitutes are available.

GET RID OF THE GLUTEN Once you've divided the food items into piles, you need to decide what to do with the gluten pile. If you're planning to keep a totally gluten-free kitchen, you can give away unopened items to neighbors or a local food shelf and toss the rest. If you're planning to keep some food items for family members that don't need to be on a gluten-free diet, you'll want to mark them carefully. It's extremely important to come up with a system you're comfortable with for keeping gluten-free and gluten-containing items completely separate in your refrigerator and pantry.

You could store gluten-free snacks and cereals on top shelves and gluten-containing versions on lower shelves. On the top shelf they're less likely to be grabbed by other family members by mistake and accidently contaminated. You could mark gluten-containing condiments and spreads with labels or stickers and corral them on the door of the refrigerator. Any system that makes cooking easy for you and keeps you, or anyone else, from accidentally mixing gluten into safe foods is a good one.

Of course, you'll need to consider the needs of your family as you establish a system. If you have a child that's gluten-free, he or she may need access to gluten-free snacks. On the flip side, if your children aren't eating gluten-free, keeping the gluten-free pretzels on a high shelf out of reach may work perfectly!

Figure out what works best for your family, and make sure everyone is in on the plan. Your gang will need to understand how you've divided the foods, so they can help keep things organized and keep everyone in the family healthy.

DO SOME CLEANING No matter how you decide to organize your kitchen, don't put anything away until you've done a good cleaning. Even tiny crumbs of gluten can be harmful to your health. You want to wash away all of the gluten hiding in the nooks and crannies of your cabinets and refrigerator so that your gluten-free foods won't become contaminated.

Remember, gluten can be messy, sticky, spongy and stubborn. Airborne flour dust and breadcrumbs can hide out in cracks and crevices. You'll want to give your kitchen a thorough cleaning before you restock it. Here are some suggestions to make sure you get rid of all of the gluten:

- **Sponges.** Buy new sponges and cleaning cloths. Your old ones may be contaminated with gluten.

- **Cabinets and cupboards.** Use a vacuum to suck up all of the loose debris and particles inside. Then wipe down all of the shelves and drawers. Don't forget the handles.

- **Refrigerator.** Wash the shelves and drawers thoroughly. And wipe off all containers before you put them back in the refrigerator.

- **Microwave and stove.** Clean your stove, cooktop and microwave. Gently scrape away caked-on foods and crumbs.

- **Oven.** Use a vacuum to suck up all of the crumbs. Then wipe down the oven walls and the racks.

- **Sink and countertops.** Always keep them clean.

If you think this sounds like a lot of work, remember you can split it up over several days. Just be sure to wash your cupboards and refrigerator before you re-shelve the food that you inventoried. Otherwise, you risk contaminating all of the food that you just sorted. You can save the stove and oven for another time, if you need to.

All of this scrubbing and scouring is worth it. Keeping a clean kitchen is important in any home. It's one of the best ways to prevent foodborne illnesses caused by common bacteria and viruses. Your need to avoid gluten is just one more reason to make sure your kitchen passes muster. You wouldn't want to eat in a restaurant that wouldn't pass a health and safety inspection. Why should it be any different in your own kitchen?

If you plan to keep some gluten-containing products in your home, you'll need to commit to regular thorough cleanings. Otherwise, flying flour dust and sprinkled crumbs can undermine your efforts to eat gluten-free.

REPLACE CONTAMINATED APPLIANCES AND UTENSILS If you've been pining for a few new items for you kitchen, you're in luck! You'll need to replace some of your cooking gear to create a gluten-safe kitchen. You don't need to dump all of your cookware and bakeware — unless you want to use your new diet as an excuse to do so! However, there are some utensils and appliances that are tough to de-gluten entirely. It's best to replace them.

Toaster If you're going to eat gluten-free breads, bagels and other toasted treats, have a gluten-free toaster. If you plan to keep gluten-containing breads in your home, keep your old toaster for these products. Purchase a new toaster for yourself. Label each toaster carefully and make sure your family understands the importance of keeping gluten-containing bread away from the designated gluten-free toaster.

Another option is to use white plastic toaster bags for toasting gluten-free bread in your regular toaster. These reusable bags protect gluten-free bread from touching any surface or element in a shared toaster.

Cutting boards Gluten may be hiding in the scratches on your cutting board. It's best to buy new ones. Choose a material that's nonporous and easy to sanitize, such as silicone. Don't buy wood or bamboo cutting boards.

If you have gluten eaters in your home, keep separate cutting boards for gluten-containing foods and for gluten-free foods. Even better, color-code them! Buy a blue cutting board for gluten-free foods and a red cutting board for foods that contain gluten. The red color is a vibrant signal that this cutting board should be avoided by anyone who needs to steer clear of gluten.

Strainer It's nearly impossible to remove gluten from all of the little holes in your strainer (colander). Start fresh with a new strainer. Again, try to buy a colored version to differentiate it from the regular strainer. Consider choosing one color — such as blue — for all of your gluten-free equipment, if possible. This can be an easy visual cue for the whole family.

Flour sifter For obvious reasons, your old flour sifter is clearly contaminated. If you plan to bake from scratch and you use a flour sifter, you'll want to invest in a new one.

Wooden spoons and other utensils Remember wood is porous and can trap small amounts of gluten. You'll want to replace wooden spoons and other wooden utensils — including salad servers and rolling pins. If you have a wooden knife block, you need to replace that, too. Carefully label your new utensils and keep them for gluten-free cooking.

Dishes, silverware, pots, pans, mixing bowls and bakeware Most of these items can simply be cleaned with hot, soapy water. However, if your cookware, bakeware, mixing bowls and other utensils are scratched or made of porous materials, they may harbor gluten particles. Cast-iron skillets and clay pizza stones also can hold gluten residue. If you're worried about residual gluten, replace those items that you feel are the most likely to harbor gluten, but you don't need to replace everything.

Other appliances Small appliances tend to be gluten hideouts. This includes your waffle iron, pancake griddle, panini maker and bread maker. If you don't think you can properly de-gluten these appliances, consider buying new ones that are reserved for gluten-free cooking.

If this list seems like a lot to purchase, don't worry. You don't have to run out and buy all of this kitchen gear right away. You might start by purchasing a cutting board, a couple of wooden spoons, a strainer and a toaster. You can buy all of these things for less than $50.

Over time, you can add to your gluten-free kitchen collection depending on the types of meals you enjoy cooking and eating the most. For example, if your family likes Saturday morning pancakes or waffles, a new waffle iron or griddle might be a good idea. You can make gluten-free versions that everyone will enjoy from a mix or from scratch. Let your tastes and culinary skills guide your decisions.

Gluten-free grocery shopping

After you get rid of all your food that contains gluten or that may contain gluten, your cupboards may look like Old Mother Hubbard's. It's time to go grocery shopping and restock your pantry and your refrigerator with a variety of delicious, gluten-free foods.

Before you head to the store, plan out your meals for the next week or the next few days and make a list of what you'll need. This way you know you'll have the right ingredients on hand. (Meal planning is discussed in the next chapter.) To make things go faster, group similar items together or organize your list according to where foods are located at your store.

When you get to the grocery store, you'll find there are far more gluten-free choices today than there were even a few years ago. In addition, the quality of gluten-free foods has improved along with the quantity. Today's gluten-free baked goods are a far cry from the cardboard-like versions that existed a decade ago.

However, it's often best to start with naturally gluten-free foods that you already know how to prepare. And then gradually add in less familiar foods and small amounts of processed gluten-free products.

This is often the recommended way to make the switch to a gluten-free diet because it gives your taste buds time to adjust to gluten-free baked goods — to forget what the regular versions of these foods taste like. In other words, you don't want to go out and buy gluten-free bread on your first shopping trip. Gluten-free breads and crackers can be delicious, but they taste different from the regular breads and crackers you're used to.

Going straight from regular bread to gluten-free bread is much like going from whole milk to skim milk or from regular soda to diet soda. Immediate comparisons aren't always favorable, but with time you learn to like them — often better.

If you can, start out eating mainly naturally gluten-free foods such as fruits, vegetables, nuts, dairy products and lean meats. And then after a month or so, begin introducing gluten-free processed foods back into your diet — items such as bread, crackers and gluten-free pizza crust.

WHERE TO SHOP All grocery stores carry hundreds of naturally gluten-free foods — foods such as fruits and vegetables, potatoes, rice, nuts and seeds, beans, fresh poultry and meat, fish, plain milk, and cheese. So no matter where you live, you'll be able to find plenty of food that you can eat at your local grocery store.

Many grocery stores also have a number of manufactured gluten-free products. Some stores have a dedicated aisle or section for gluten-free foods. Others stock gluten-free offerings in the health food section or specialties aisle. Some keep gluten-free products alongside their traditional counterparts — for example, putting gluten-free flours in the baking aisle. You'll also find gluten-free foods in the freezer case and refrigerator section. Some stores have printed guides to help you easily locate all of their gluten-free products.

Depending on where you live, you might find everything you need at your regular supermarket. Or you may need to head to a larger grocery store in a neighboring city or to a nearby natural foods store or cooperative.

Identify one or two or three stores where you can easily accomplish the bulk of your grocery shopping, and stick with them. If you're a regular patron at a particular store, you'll become familiar with the available gluten-free foods and where they're located in the store. This is much more efficient than searching for gluten-free products in an unfamiliar store every week.

To help you get started, here are some gluten-free staples you might want to add to your shopping list:

Fruits and vegetables
Fresh fruits
Fresh vegetables
Potatoes
Frozen vegetables
(no sauce)
Frozen fruits
Canned vegetables
(no sauce)
Tomato sauce
Tomato paste
Dried fruits

Grains
Rice (white, brown, wild)
Naturally gluten-free
grains (see page 177)
Gluten-free oatmeal
Gluten-free cereals
Gluten-free bread
Gluten-free pasta
Corn tortillas and
taco shells

Meats and protein
Meat, poultry and fish
Canned tuna
Beans (black, kidney,
garbanzo)
Unseasoned nuts and
peanut butter

Dairy
Milk
Eggs
Gluten-free yogurt
Cheese
Cottage cheese

Other
Vegetable and olive oil
Plain herbs and spices
Gluten-free chicken broth
Gluten-free mayonnaise,
mustard, ketchup and
BBQ sauce
Jelly, jam and honey
Olives and pickles
Salsa and gluten-free
corn chips
Plain popcorn
Plain ice cream and
frozen yogurt

Keep in mind that you can also purchase gluten-free foods online from gluten-free bakeries and millers, large manufacturers, and large retailers. Online shopping may be particularly helpful if you live in a small town and the local grocery store doesn't carry a lot of gluten-free products.

Farmers markets can be an inexpensive source of fresh, local, naturally gluten-free products — including fruits, veggies, herbs, specialty cheeses, meat, free-range eggs, honey, maple syrup and other goods. But be cautious about buying baked goods and prepared foods. Although some venders may sell gluten-free items such as breads and cookies, these items won't be labeled. You'll have to determine how reliable the vender is and whether there could be any cross-contamination. If you have any doubt about a product, skip it.

HOW TO SHOP If you typically wander up and down every aisle in the store when you shop for groceries, you may need to forge a new shopping strategy. It can be confusing and defeating to weave your way through aisle after aisle of questionable products. Instead, you want to spend your time where most of the gluten-free goods are located.

Stick to the perimeter Focus your attention on the perimeter of the grocery store. Purchasing most of your food from the perimeter of the store is a good strategy for healthy eating in general. It's particularly important when you're on the hunt for gluten-free foods.

The produce, dairy, meat and seafood sections of most grocery stores are all located on the perimeter. Most of these fresh foods are naturally gluten-free. These foods are better for you than ready-to-eat foods because you can control the ingredients that you add.

If you're not an expert in the kitchen, start with the basics — foods such as fresh vegetables and fruit, potatoes, cheese and eggs, and fresh meat and poultry. Over time, you can experiment with more unusual fruits, vegetables, meats and seafood.

Spend time in the gluten-free section After you've stocked up on the basics, make your way to the store's gluten-free section. There you'll find pastas, cereals and snacks. Be sure to look at the labels on the products you purchase to make sure they're not loaded with sugar or fat. Soon you'll become familiar with the foods in this section, and you'll know right away which ones fit your diet.

Be selective in the center aisles Check your list. Remember those items you threw out? These are the ones you'll want to find gluten-free substitutes for.

Some of these items may be located in the gluten-free section. Others may be shelved with their gluten-containing counterparts in the center aisles.

Read every food label As you learned in Chapter 13, it's important to check every label for gluten, even the labels of products that you've purchased before. Manufacturers can change the ingredients at any time, so you need to double-check every label and ingredient list each time you buy a product.

Don't shop when you're hungry You've probably heard this tip before, and it applies to a gluten-free diet, too. Shopping when you're hungry can make it more difficult to resist items that you shouldn't eat. If you're famished, you may also hurry through the store rather than taking time to read food labels carefully. You're more likely to make mistakes and overlook hidden sources of gluten if you're rushing.

It's best to shop after you've eaten a good meal. If you do find yourself shopping on an empty stomach, drink some water or buy a piece of fresh fruit to munch on while you shop.

An easy on-the-go option

We all have them, those days when you're particularly busy or perhaps you're traveling and you don't have time to sit down and eat, so you eat on the run. If you need to avoid gluten, grabbing something in a hurry can be even more difficult.

One way to handle such situations is to carry with you meal replacement beverages such as Ensure. These products are generally gluten-free, and they're healthy. They can be a lifesaver when you're hungry or you need a quick snack and you don't have time to find something to eat.

Be prepared to spend a few hours on your first few trips to the grocery store. (Many people spend the better part of an afternoon at the grocery store on their first venture.) If you're prepared for this, it won't seem as bad. Keep in mind that you don't have to fill your grocery cart on that first shopping trip. Just buy the essentials — enough to get you through a few days.

Grocery shopping won't always be a lengthy chore. Before long, you'll be accustomed to the gluten-free foods at your favorite stores, and your shopping trips will be back to their usual time frame.

Your store navigator

To give you an at-a-glance look for how to shop, here's a layout of a grocery store. Your store may be configured a little differently, but the same basic principles apply. Follow the footsteps. They indicate the areas of the store that contain the most gluten-free foods.

Fruits and vegetables. The more time you spend here, the better! All fresh fruits and vegetables are naturally gluten-free. Fill your cart with a bounty of seasonal produce.

Bakery. It's probably best to avoid the bakery. Assume that all items there contain gluten.

Bulk bins. Many of the ingredients in the organic bulk bins could be perfect for a gluten-free diet. Unfortunately, there's a high risk of cross-contamination in this section. Shoppers may innocently use the same scoop they used to gather white flour to purchase some gluten-free buckwheat. So it's best to avoid the bulk bins entirely. Instead, buy pre-packed versions of these items.

Meat and seafood. Fresh meat, fish and seafood are excellent gluten-free choices. Buy plain cuts — no stuffed, breaded, marinated or pre-basted varieties. Poultry that's labeled as "pre-basted" or "self-basting" may contain a marinade and may not be gluten-free. Meat and fish substitutes, such as vegetarian burgers or mock duck may include seitan, another word for wheat gluten. Products made from ground fish may contain wheat starch and other gluten-containing flavorings. It's best to purchase real fish, not imitation varieties.

Packaged meats. Some processed deli meats, salami, hot dogs and bacon contain fillers or barley flavoring agents. Ask questions and check labels at the deli counter. If your store doesn't have a dedicated gluten-free slicer, stick to gluten-free packaged deli meats to avoid cross-contamination.

Dairy. The dairy case is generally a safe zone unless you have trouble digesting lactose. One exception is flavored yogurts. Some have gluten-containing ingredients or granolas added to them. Also check the labels on cheese sauces and flavored cream cheeses. Some have gluten-containing fillers or flavoring agents.

Organic and ethnic foods. Make sure to read the labels. Just because a product is made from organic ingredients doesn't mean it's gluten-free. If you're not sure what some of the ingredients in ethnic foods are, it's best not to purchase those items.

Packaged goods. In general, limit the time you spend here. Read the labels on everything. Good choices here include rice, beans, unseasoned nuts and gluten-free nut butters, gluten-free breakfast cereals, and plain popcorn. Beware that some condiments contain gluten. Plain versions of dried herbs and spices are best. Mixed blends and packets may contain gluten.

Frozen foods. Plain frozen fruits and vegetables without sauces are great gluten-free choices. Also look for plain frozen poultry, meat and seafood, as well as frozen ice cream and yogurt. In some stores, the freezer section is where you'll find gluten-free frozen bread and pie crusts and gluten-free pizza. To be safe, read all labels carefully.

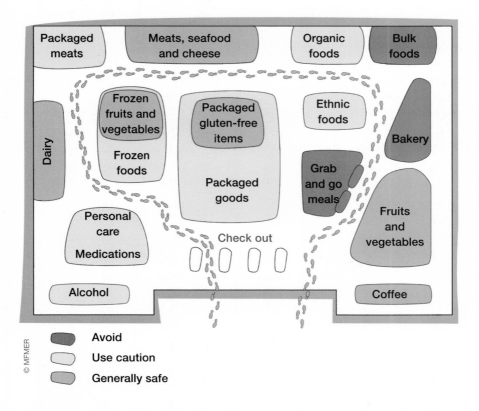

© MFMER

Avoid

Use caution

Generally safe

Cutting costs

As you may already know, some gluten-free foods are expensive. Fresh produce, meat and fish can be pricey. In addition, gluten-free flours, breads, cereals, cookies, pastas and snacks often cost three to five times more than the traditional versions.

There's a reason for the price difference. In order to produce gluten-free foods, manufacturers typically buy gluten-free grains such as rice, corn or buckwheat from farmers and millers who take special precautions to ensure that the grains aren't contaminated during the harvesting and shipping processes. This often comes at a premium price. In addition, manufacturers have to pay for dedicated equipment, processing techniques and testing to ensure that their products are gluten-free. These costs all trickle down to the supermarket shelves.

On the flip side, a gluten-free diet can result in some cost savings. When you eat gluten-free, you generally aren't purchasing as many processed and prepared foods, which tend to be more expensive. You may also find that you don't eat out at restaurants as often or purchase as much takeout food as you used to. This can also save you money.

MONEY-SAVING STRATEGIES Here are a few suggestions on ways that you can eat well and save money on a gluten-free diet:

Plan your meals Decide what meals you're going to make in the coming week and put together a shopping list of what you'll need. This way you won't buy food that you won't need.

Think seasonal Purchase fruits and vegetables in season when they're at their peak in flavor and generally at their bottom in price. A neighborhood farmers market can be an excellent source of reasonably priced fresh, great-tasting local produce.

Bake from scratch Gluten-free baked goods sold in stores, such as those found at specialty bakeries, can be expensive. Try baking your own instead. At first, you may need to buy a lot of gluten-free ingredients, and they aren't as cheap as the traditional versions. So the initial cost may seem unreasonable. But if you bake regularly, you'll quickly recoup your investment.

Go with the basics Serve rice, especially brown rice, and potatoes for side dishes most of the time. Save more expensive gluten-free pastas for special occasions. In general, limiting the number of processed gluten-free products you purchase will help your budget.

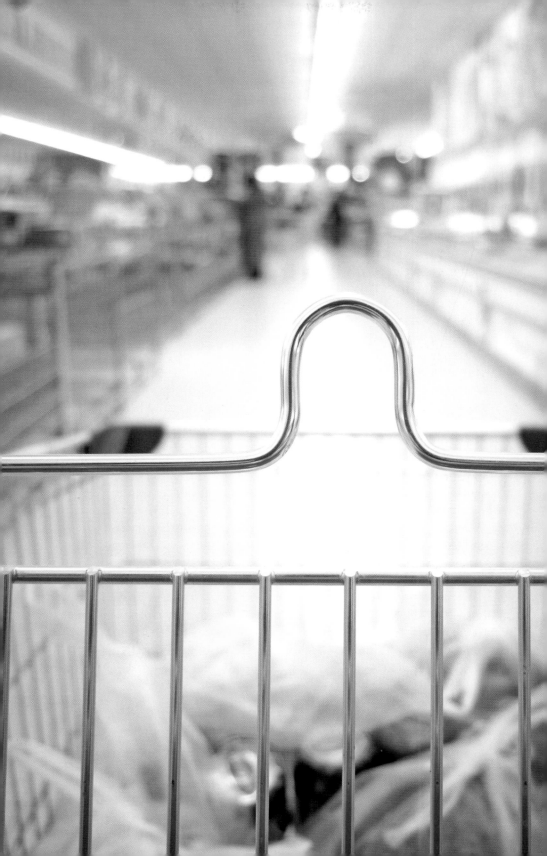

Try samples Before you invest in a lot of expensive gluten-free products, see if you can taste test them first to determine if you like them. Gluten-free samples are sometimes available at gluten-free or celiac disease events. Some manufacturers also offer sampler packs or variety packs. Many are available online.

Buy in bulk Once you find gluten-free products that you like, buying in bulk can save you money. You can purchase breads, baking mixes and snacks in economy sizes, or even in cases at warehouse clubs and online retailers. You can store or freeze perishable gluten-free items for future use if you can't eat them right away.

Be a smart snacker Limit the amount of gluten-free crackers, cookies and other snacks that you purchase. And remember, when you do buy more expensive gluten-free snacks, you don't need to share them with family members who can eat cheaper versions that contain gluten.

Use coupons and flyers Look for gluten-free product coupons online. Also take advantage of frequent shopper cards and rewards programs at your local stores.

Apply for a tax deduction Find out if you can write off certain expenses associated with your diet. You may be able to deduct the excess cost of gluten-free foods if you have to follow a gluten-free diet for medical reasons. If you qualify for a tax deduction, you'll need to submit an official written diagnosis from your doctor with your tax records. You'll also have to submit receipts for all of your gluten-free groceries along with a record of the deductible differ-ence between the gluten-free groceries that you purchased and the regular versions. This can be extremely time-consuming, but for some people it's worth the effort.

If you're struggling to eat gluten-free because of the added expense, talk to your dietitian. He or she can help you plan meals that are within your budget. Whatever you do, don't cut corners on your health. If a gluten-free diet can help you feel better and stay healthy, the added expense is worth it.

Time to start cooking!

In the next chapter, we'll talk about how to cook and bake without gluten. As you just read, one way to save money is to prepare most of your foods yourself instead of buying processed versions or eating out at restaurants. Gluten-free cooking isn't as difficult as you may think. Sure, there may be a period of trial and error, but with time you'll learn how to prepare a number of foods — foods you may have thought you'd never eat again! Just because you can't have gluten doesn't mean that you can't enjoy some delicious food, such as a warm gluten-free brownie!

CHAPTER FIFTEEN

Cooking without gluten

Grilled rib-eye steak. Spicy black bean chili. Sliced watermelon. Perfect baked ham. Flourless chocolate cake. Broiled salmon. Wild rice casserole. Steamed asparagus. Mango sorbet. Guacamole with corn tortilla chips. Scrambled eggs. Garlic mashed potatoes. Crunchy apples with caramel dip. Homemade chicken tenders. Tasty trail mix. Chef's salad.

All of these foods are either naturally gluten-free or they can be made without gluten. They're just the beginning of your gluten-free adventure!

In the preceding chapter, you learned how to restock your pantry with healthy, gluten-free staples. This chapter shows you how to turn those hard-earned ingredients into delicious meals. Keeping to the key principles that you learned in earlier chapters, this chapter focuses on learning how to cook without gluten in a simple manner. You'll learn how to start with familiar ingredients and recipes and gradually expand your cooking skills from there. Even if you've never cooked, you can learn how to do it.

As you've read, preparing meals in your own kitchen is generally the best way to begin a gluten-free diet. Cooking at home gives you control over exactly what goes into your food and how it's prepared. It also helps you avoid hidden gluten and cross-contamination. Creating new and tasty meals will not only help heal your body but also can be a fun experience. You'll learn that with the right attitude and ingredients you can still eat the foods you enjoy.

Getting started

Cooking and baking from scratch can alleviate some of the challenges of gluten-free living. When you dine at home, you can avoid the confused waiter who delivers your gluten-free salad topped with croutons. You can enjoy a meal with friends without worrying about hidden ingredients. You can eat warm, gluten-free bread or oozing, gluten-free chocolate chip cookies straight from the oven. And you may find a sense of accomplishment in taking the reins and cooking your way to good health.

If you're worried because you don't like to cook or you worry that you're not a skilled cook, that's OK. Gluten-free cooking doesn't require special talent, advanced skills, complicated recipes, fancy pots or hours in front of a hot stove. You can make unfussy gluten-free meals with a crockpot, grill or microwave that involve simple ingredients and minimal time and effort.

If you don't cook at all or if you cook very little, you may need to learn some basic cooking techniques, but these are skills you can easily master. Start out with meals that require only two or three ingredients and take just a matter of minutes to prepare. Move on to more involved recipes when you feel ready. You can find thousands of recipe ideas in cookbooks and online.

Learning to cook without gluten is a step-by-step process.

❋ To start, focus on naturally gluten-free foods that you already know how to make, whether that's a grilled steak or a green salad.

❋ Next, move on to meals that require simple substitutions to become gluten-free. For example, if your family likes meatloaf or macaroni and cheese, you can make it gluten-free.

❋ When you feel comfortable in your new role, start experimenting with uncommon gluten-free grains, more challenging gluten-free recipes and further adaptations of your favorite recipes. You'll find cooking and substitution tips throughout this chapter to help you.

Cooking without gluten starts with good-quality, fresh ingredients and a few basic cooking techniques that anyone can master. Even if cooking isn't your passion, with a little time and practice you can become quite proficient. You'll be amazed at what you can create in your own kitchen with a little extra effort!

PLAN YOUR WEEK The first step in gluten-free cooking is to plan your meals for the week. As you learned in Chapter 14, creating a weekly menu can have a big impact on your health — and your budget. Thinking ahead helps ensure that you have the right ingredients on hand when cooking. Meal planning can also cut your grocery costs by minimizing food waste and expensive last-minute takeout meals.

Smart meal planning is a timesaver, too. It can cut down on unplanned trips to the grocery store to buy one or two items. Plus, you can save time by prepping ingredients, such as chopping vegetables, for multiple meals at once. Or you can use leftovers from one meal in another.

To get started, make a list of all the meals you normally eat that are naturally gluten-free. This includes breakfasts, lunches and dinners, as well as some desserts. And don't forget about snacks. If you enjoy cottage cheese with fresh strawberries or prepared hummus with veggies, you're already snacking gluten-free. If you typically grab breakfast and lunch on the go, a dietitian can give you a list of simple recipes to get you started.

Next, add in family favorites that could easily be turned into gluten-free meals with one or two modifications. For example, if your family likes spaghetti with meat and tomato sauce, just swap out the regular pasta for gluten-free pasta. If tacos are a tradition at your house, make sure to use gluten-free corn tortillas or shells instead of the wheat variety and check the ingredients on the taco mix to make sure it doesn't include gluten.

When you have breakfast, lunch and dinner mapped out for the upcoming week, along with some snacks, start compiling your grocery list. You may need to carefully review your recipes to make sure you've included everything you need on your list. Make sure to check your cupboard or refrigerator to see if you already have some of the items you'll need. You'll know you're getting pretty good at meal planning when you can do all, or most, of your grocery shopping for the week in a single trip.

Here are some things to consider as you plan your meals:

❋ **Know your schedule.** If you typically eat out on Friday night, scratch that meal off your list. If you have to work late or you have a commitment on a certain night, pencil in leftovers or a meal that you can quickly prepare and serve. If you have an early exercise class on Tuesday morning, plan a simple breakfast that you can carry with you. Make sure your menu plans fit with your weekly schedule.

❋ **Take inventory.** Survey your kitchen cupboards and refrigerator before deciding on your weekly menus. It may spark your imagination.

❋ **Think seasonal.** What fresh produce is available this time of year? Is it salad season or soup weather? Changing your menus with the seasons is typically healthier and cheaper.

* **Aim for variety.** Different kinds of food contain different nutrients. When you eat a wide variety, there's a greater likelihood that you're getting all the recommended amounts of vitamins and minerals you need for good health. Plus, you're less likely to get bored with your diet.

* **Avoid ruts.** It's easy to get into a rut and make the same thing over and over. This is especially true if your list of gluten-free recipes isn't very long. Try to be creative. A smoothie is an easy and delicious lunch or snack. You can also designate theme nights — such as meatless Mondays or fish Fridays or soup Sundays — and see what new ideas you can come up with.

* **Plan for leftovers.** Leftovers can be a lifesaver. Consider making a large pot of stew on the weekend so that you have some for lunch during the week. Or grill a batch of chicken breasts on Saturday or Sunday so that you have leftover meat to make chicken salad, chicken wraps or chicken and rice soup for lunch. These dishes can also be quick dinners for busy nights.

* **Use certain foods first.** Fresh vegetables and fruits should be eaten at the beginning of the week and frozen varieties later in the week. That way you can avoid throwing away expensive produce that's past its prime. Some fresh vegetables and fruits have shorter shelf lives than others. Factor this into your meal planning.

* **Consider the whole family.** If some members of your family prefer food that contains gluten, think about how you can accommodate their tastes without making two separate meals. You can make gluten-free meals that everyone will love, such as grilled flank steak or chicken and cheddar quesadillas with corn tortillas. Another option is to make a gluten-free main dish but with two serving options. You can serve barbecued pulled pork on regular buns for your family and place it on top of potatoes for yourself.

Let your personal preferences and lifestyle guide some of your decisions. As you may have realized, eating gluten-free is a bit of a learning curve. Thinking ahead with a good menu plan can increase your confidence and keep you on track.

EXPAND YOUR HORIZONS Once you're in the rhythm of menu planning and meal preparation, challenge yourself to new recipes. Look for recipes that are enticing in addition to being gluten-free — meals that you look forward to trying. If you're still not real confident in the kitchen, aim for simple recipes with two or three main ingredients and preparation times of 20 minutes or less.

There are many excellent gluten-free cookbooks and online recipe resources. Or skip the cookbooks and experiment freestyle with the knowledge you already have. Improvise with different flavors and ingredients that appeal to your taste buds. Expect an occasional mishap when you go off recipe. That's OK. But in general, it's hard to go wrong if you start with good-quality ingredients and prepare them simply.

Don't be afraid to test out new fruits and vegetables, legumes, and meat cuts that you've never cooked before. You can even experiment with a range of flavors, textures and colors. You may need to use a recipe when you cook new ingredients for the first time. But you'll be amazed at the number of recipes you can find for these less common foods.

In addition to experimenting with new ingredients, try different cooking techniques. Perhaps you don't care for baking, but you might enjoy stir-frying or grilling. Braising and poaching are worth trying, too. These cooking methods impart a lot of flavor without adding excessive amounts of fat.

Recipe makeovers

You can find thousands of gluten-free recipes in cookbooks and online, but you'll probably want to prepare your own recipes — favorites that have been served on your family's table for decades. Sometimes, these cherished recipes

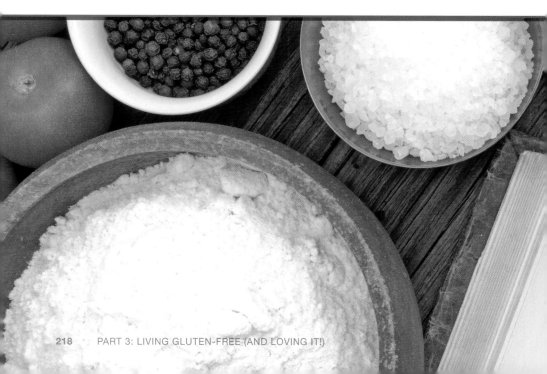

have one or two key ingredients that contain gluten. You may feel deprived if you have to give them up, which only makes you crave the food even more.

Fortunately, almost any recipe can be adapted to become gluten-free. It may take a little creativity and experimentation with ingredients you've never tried before, but you'll get there. Some won't taste exactly like the original recipe. But your gluten-free version can be equally delicious.

To begin with, identify those ingredients that contain gluten. Sometimes, you can simply substitute gluten-free versions of those ingredients. For example, you might make your grandmother's stuffing recipe with gluten-free bread or cornbread and gluten-free chicken broth. Other times, you may need to adjust the ingredients and the cooking times.

Carefully review your recipe, and mark any items that you think can be omitted or substituted. Check gluten-free cookbooks or websites for the best gluten-free substitutes. If your recipe includes a lot of packaged, store-bought products, such as sauces, marinades or dry mixes, you might be able to replace them with brands that are gluten-free or with versions you make from scratch.

As you swap ingredients in your regular recipes, focus on re-creating the prominent flavors. Sometimes, the texture is important, too. If you eliminate the coating because it contains gluten, you may need to find another way to add crunch. Also be aware that gluten-free baked goods often require adjusting the other ingredients in the recipe, for example, the number of eggs, to achieve the same texture and flavor as the original recipe.

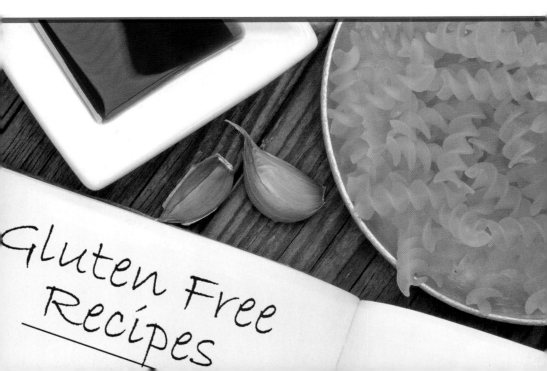

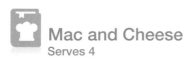

Mac and Cheese
Serves 4

Dietitian's tip: It's easy to overcook gluten-free pasta so that it turns mushy. To cook it properly, bring the water to a rolling boil and then add the uncooked pasta. Set the timer for about 3 minutes less than the recommended cooking time on the package. Test the pasta when the timer goes off and every minute after until it's perfectly cooked. Then drain and rinse with cold water right away.

Ingredients	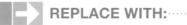 REPLACE WITH:
» 12 ounces uncooked elbow macaroni	**12 ounces uncooked (brown rice) elbow macaroni**
» 3½ cups milk*, divided	
» 4 tablespoons flour	**2 tablespoons cornstarch**
» 4 tablespoons butter	
» ½ teaspoon salt*	
» 8 ounces (2 cups) cheddar cheese, shredded	
» 2 ounces (½ cup) Parmesan cheese, grated	
» ½ cup breadcrumbs	**½ cup gluten-free breadcrumbs – (or gluten-free panko-style crumbs)**
» Paprika, black or cayenne pepper – to taste	

*Milk and salt are gluten-free. There is already plenty of fat and sodium in the cheeses, so you can lower the fat content by using lower fat milk and lower the sodium content by omitting the salt.

1. Preheat oven to 400 F.
2. In a large pot, cook the gluten-free rice pasta according to package directions. (Do not overcook pasta.) Drain pasta in strainer, rinse with cold water to stop cooking. Shake pasta while rinsing to keep it from clumping. Set aside.
3. In a small bowl, mix half the milk with the cornstarch.
4. In the empty pot, melt butter over medium heat. Whisk in the remaining milk and bring to a simmer. Continue to whisk while adding the cornstarch mixture. Continue to cook over medium heat while sauce thickens, about 5 minutes. Add the cheeses and continue to stir until melted. Add seasonings.
5. Stir pasta into sauce. Pour into 2-quart baking dish. Sprinkle with breadcrumbs.
6. Bake 15 minutes — or until browned. Cool 5 minutes and serve.

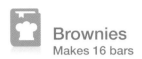

Brownies
Makes 16 bars

Dietitian's tip: These brownies are fudgy and moist — not runny or dry. To make them, you'll need the basic gluten-free flour mix recipe on page 224.

Ingredients	REPLACE WITH:

» 1 cup (2 sticks) butter, cut into chunks ····· **12 tablespoons (1½ sticks) butter, cut into chunks**

» 2 cups sugar ·································· **1½ cups sugar**

» ½ cup unsweetened cocoa powder ········ **¾ cup unsweetened cocoa powder**

» ½ teaspoon salt

» 2 large eggs

» 1 teaspoon vanilla extract

» 1½ cups flour ································ **¾ cup gluten-free flour mix**

» ⅔ cup chopped walnuts (optional)

1. Position the oven rack in the lower third of the oven. Preheat oven to 350 F.

2. Line an 8-inch square baking pan with foil or parchment paper. (To help remove brownies from pan, leave an extra amount of foil or paper overhanging on opposite sides.)

3. Fill a medium-sized saucepan half full with water and bring to a simmer. Put butter chunks, sugar, cocoa powder and salt in a large heatproof bowl. Place bowl over simmering water. Stir while butter melts and mixture warms, about 5 minutes.

4. Remove bowl from heat and set aside.

5. In a separate bowl, whisk together eggs and vanilla. Add to cooled chocolate mixture. Add flour and stir well to combine. (Add walnuts if desired.)

6. Scrape batter into prepared pan and smooth with back of spatula.

7. Bake for 15 minutes. Insert a toothpick into the center. If still runny, rotate pan and bake another 10 to 15 minutes. Repeat until toothpick comes out with moist crumbs.

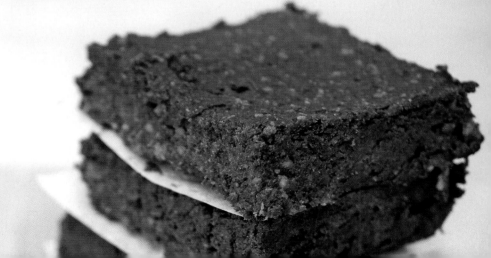

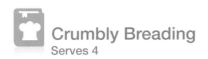 **Crumbly Breading**
Serves 4

Dietitian's tip: Each breadcrumb substitute has a slightly different flavor and texture. Shrimp pairs well with neutral-flavored, gluten-free panko-style breadcrumbs. Fish goes well with gluten-free crackers. Chicken is a good match for crushed gluten-free cornflakes. For pork, gluten-free breadcrumbs are a nice choice; they're a bit heavier and blend well with seasonings such as sage. If you're in a hurry, you can use crushed gluten-free rice crackers with any meat or seafood. They're an easy breading to keep on hand.

Ingredients	REPLACE WITH:

» 1 pound chicken tenders, pork fillets, fish or shrimp

» Salt and pepper, and other herbs and spices to taste

» 2 eggs

» 2 cups breadcrumbs ·················· **Choose 2 cups of any of the following:**
- **Gluten-free breadcrumbs**
- **Gluten-free panko-style breadcrumbs**
- **Gluten-free cornflakes (crushed)**
- **Gluten-free crackers (crushed)**

» ½ cup all-purpose flour ··············· **½ cup cornstarch**

» ½ cup milk ····························· **Omit**

1. Preheat oven to 375 F.
2. Season meat or fish with salt and pepper.
3. In a shallow dish, beat eggs and set aside.
4. Place crumbs into second shallow dish. Add seasonings if desired (see seasoning options below).
5. Place cornstarch into large plastic bag.
6. Pat meat or fish dry with paper towels. Add one or two pieces or fillets to plastic bag and shake the bag to coat evenly. Remove from bag, shaking off excess cornstarch.
7. Dip meat or fish into beaten eggs, then press and roll in crumbs to coat evenly.
8. Place on baking sheet. Repeat until all pieces are breaded.
9. Bake in oven for about 15 minutes or until golden brown.

Seasoning options: Add about ¼ teaspoon of one of the ingredients below to the breading mixture to lightly season it. Add more if you prefer a stronger taste.

» Garlic powder	» Cayenne pepper	» Rosemary
» Onion powder	» Lemon pepper or zest	» Oregano
» Ginger powder	» Paprika	» Mustard powder

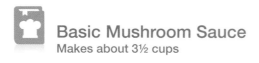

Basic Mushroom Sauce
Makes about 3½ cups

Dietitian's tip: Use this sauce in place of a gluten-filled gravy or as a substitute for canned creamed soup in casseroles or other recipes. Adding gluten-free rice flour to the mushrooms, onion and oil creates a roux (pronounced roo). The roux helps thicken the sauce while keeping the flour from clumping when the liquid is added. Be sure to add the liquids gradually, and don't let the mixture boil or it will scald.

Ingredients	REPLACE WITH:

- » 8 ounces (about 3 cups) sliced mushrooms
- » ¼ cup chopped onion
- » 1 tablespoon olive oil
- » ¼ cup flour ·································· **¼ cup gluten-free rice flour**
- » 2 cups chicken broth ··················· **2 cups gluten-free chicken broth**
- » 1 cup milk
- » ½ teaspoon salt
- » Black pepper, to taste
- » Herb of choice: thyme, chives, rosemary or tarragon

1. In a 3-quart saucepan over medium heat, stir and sauté mushrooms and onion with olive oil until onions are translucent and mushrooms give off moisture.
2. Sprinkle with gluten-free flour and continue to stir mixture for another 2 to 3 minutes.
3. Add gluten-free chicken broth and then milk. Continue to cook over medium heat until thickened. Season with salt, pepper and desired herbs.

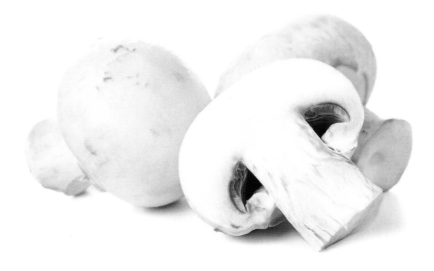

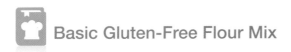

Basic Gluten-Free Flour Mix

Dietitian's tip: This flour mixture may be used in place of flour made from wheat in cookies, muffins, pancakes or crepes.

Ingredients

» 3 cups rice flour
» 3 cups potato starch flour
» 1 cup cornstarch

1. Lightly spoon rice flour into measuring cup. When mounded, use the flat edge of a knife to level the flour. Pour into large bowl.
2. Repeat with potato starch flour and cornstarch.
3. Whisk together to combine, then store in either airtight container or self-locking plastic bag. Keep in cool, dark location.

Basic substitutions

Here are a few common substitutions that may come in handy as you give your old recipes a gluten-free face-lift:

If your recipes call for:	Use instead:
All-purpose flour	» Basic gluten-free flour mix (see above)
Bread in stuffing	» Gluten-free cornbread
	» Rice or wild rice
	» Quinoa
Breadcrumb toppings on casseroles	» Crushed corn chips or potato chips
	» Crushed gluten-free finely chopped nuts
Flour to thicken gravy	» Arrowroot starch flour
	» Cornstarch
	» Tapioca starch
	» Sweet rice flour
Flour in puddings or pie fillings	» Arrowroot starch flour
	» Cornstarch
	» Tapioca flour
Flour in white sauce or roux	» Sweet rice flour
	» Cornstarch
	» Tapioca starch

Gluten-free baking

Once you get the knack of gluten-free cooking, give yourself a chance to stretch your growing culinary skills. Consider making your own gluten-free breads, cookies and other baked goods. Gluten-free baking takes some willingness to experiment and you can expect occasional misfires, but you can make gluten-free baked goods that are much cheaper — and tastier — than store-bought versions. Plus, there's nothing like the taste of hot, homemade cookies from your own oven.

FLOUR Gluten-free baking may seem complicated at first. That's because a single gluten-free flour is rarely a good stand-in for the traditional stuff. For the best results, you want to mix three or four gluten-free flours together to substitute for basic all-purpose flour. In addition, every gluten-free flour has a different taste and texture. Some are ideally suited for pizza dough and savory scones. Some are best for breads such as muffins and pancakes. And others are suited for yeast breads. There truly is no best "all-purpose" gluten-free flour.

That's where experimentation comes in. You'll want to test different combinations of gluten-free flours to learn how to take advantage of their natural traits. Gluten-free cookbooks and websites can help guide you. Remember, a good flour mix can provide you with more than just the basis for bread. The mixture may also serve well as breading or coating for meat and as a thickener for broths, gravies and stews. For more on gluten-free flours, see page 229.

If this sounds like too much work and you prefer to keep it simple, there are gluten-free baking mixes that you can purchase that don't require you to blend your own flours. It's all done for you. You substitute them cup for cup in any recipe that calls for wheat flour.

OTHER INGREDIENTS Gluten-free flour isn't the only component of gluten-free baking. You'll also need to learn how to adjust other ingredients in the recipe, such as oil and eggs, when you use gluten-free flours. If you're using a drier flour, you may need additional liquids to keep the food moist.

In addition, you may want to add xantham gum (see page 226). This gluten-free baking ingredient helps gluten-free flours mimic the effects of regular flour. It binds the ingredients together and provides leavening and texture. Xantham gum is available at some grocery stores, health foods stores and mail-order companies.

A FEW TIPS Baking times can also take a bit of trial and error. When using gluten-free starches and flours, you often need to bake the items a bit longer and at a lower temperature than what's called for in the original recipe.

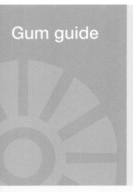

Gum guide

If a recipe states how much xantham gum to add, follow the recipe. If you're modifying an existing recipe, here's the general rule of thumb for how much xantham gum to include.

Food	Amount of xantham gum
Bread and pizza dough	1 teaspoon gum per cup of flour
Cakes, muffins, quick breads	½ teaspoon gum per cup of flour
Cookies and bars	½ teaspoon or less per cup of flour

Over time, you'll become familiar with the science of gluten-free baking, but at first it takes a little patience. In general, recipes that contain pureed fruit, yogurt or sour cream, such as banana bread or pumpkin muffins, tend to translate to gluten-free more easily than do cakes and cookies that rely primarily on flour. You might want to start with more forgiving recipes, then try more complicated recipes as your comfort level and confidence increase.

If you bake your own bread, you may want to purchase a bread machine. It can take some of the guesswork out of gluten-free baking. You can find bread machines with a gluten-free cycle, but it may be just as effective to use a rapid cycle with a single rise. (Gluten-free breads don't require two rises.) No matter what type of machine or cycle you choose, a good recipe or mix is still important.

Avoiding cross-contamination

When you're cooking and baking, be very careful to prevent gluten cross-contamination in your home. As you learned in the previous chapter, if some members of your family eat gluten products, you'll need to develop a system for storing your gluten-free foods and ingredients separately from those that contain gluten.

Also be careful not to share utensils, pots and pans, and baking equipment without washing them thoroughly. For certain utensils and appliances, such as toasters, grinders, sifters, and measuring cups and spoons, it's best to have two of them or two sets — one used only for gluten-free foods and the other for foods containing gluten.

Here are some other tips to help prevent cross-contamination in your kitchen:

❋ **Wash your hands.** Wash them frequently with soap. Make sure your family members get sudsy, too.

Clean as you go. Wipe off surfaces before you put your food down and after you're done preparing food. Teach your family members to do the same. You don't want crumbs from your son's peanut butter and jelly sandwich on the counter when you start making your gluten-free cookies.

Don't double-dip. Make sure no one in your house dips a knife into butter or condiments after the knife has touched regular bread or other gluten-containing foods. This common mistake contaminates the entire stick of butter or jar of mustard. The same is true of measuring cups and spoons that dip between regular flour and gluten-free baking ingredients.

Create a barrier. When grilling, place your chicken, meat or fish on tinfoil, rather than placing it directly on the grill rack. This trick works for many roasting and baking recipes, too. The tinfoil creates a barrier between your gluten-free food and any gluten that is stuck to the cooking surface.

Some people mistakenly believe that gluten will cook away or be killed off at high temperatures. But that's not true. The only way to remove gluten is to wash it away. Keep cleaning supplies handy so that you can easily wipe off countertops and utensils and get back to creating tasty gluten-free foods.

Some simple cooking strategies

Remember, you don't have to be a gourmet chef to be a good home cook. By devoting just a little more time and commitment to the task of preparing meals, you may be pleasantly surprised at what you can accomplish. These strategies can help set you up for success:

Plan ahead as much as possible. This way you'll always have the right ingredients on hand for what you're trying to prepare. Use extras and leftovers to reduce your time in the kitchen.

Make sure you have the proper equipment. You don't need a lot of expensive, fancy gear, but you'll want some basic, good-quality cooking tools.

Organize your kitchen in a way that works for you. Make sure to separate foods that don't contain gluten from those that do.

- ❋ **Use shortcuts.** This includes prepackaged salad greens (with no dressing) and pre-cut carrots. Keep gluten-free canned soups and other prepared items in your pantry for days that you don't have a lot of time to cook.

- ❋ **Don't always use the oven.** To save time, experiment with convenient cooking techniques, including using a slow cooker or your microwave.

- ❋ **Take advantage of your freezer.** Buy in bulk or make double batches and divide items into smaller quantities that you can thaw and cook for one or two meals. Freezing keeps food fresh longer and helps prevent waste.

- ❋ **Look for flavorful ingredients.** Fresh herbs and plain spices are gluten-free, and they can add color, taste and aroma. Sharp cheeses, olives, sun-dried tomatoes, bacon and other pungent ingredients can also add big flavor to your meals, even if you only use a small amount.

In the end, preparing your own meals can be pleasurable. Many people find that it gives them a sense of control over their health. Cooking doesn't need to be drudgery.

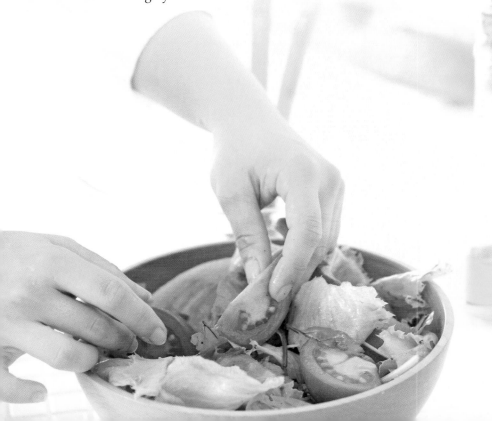

Glossary of gluten-free flours

You can find many of these gluten-free flours in supermarkets. If these products aren't available at your local grocery store, look for them online or at a health foods store.

Each gluten-free flour has different desirable properties. You often need to combine three or four gluten-free flours to make a mix for gluten-free baking. Here's a sampling of options and how to use them.

Amaranth flour

This flour has a nutty, slightly sweet, toasted flavor. Try it in baked goods that are dark in color, such as brownies or spiced treats.

Arrowroot starch flour

This is a good substitute for cornstarch. It can be used for breading, as a thickener for fruit sauces or blended with other gluten-free flours to make baked goods.

Bean flour

Made from various ground, dried beans — such as navy, pinto, black, cranberry, fava, chickpea (garbanzo), soy and white beans — bean flours pair well with sorghum flour in recipes with intense flavors, such as gingerbread and chocolate cake.

Corn flour

Milled from ground corn kernels, corn flour has a light texture, and it gives baked goods a slightly nutty flavor. It's not as coarse as cornmeal.

Mesquite flour

Available in a coarse meal or a fine flour, this flour has a slightly sweet, chocolate, molasses-like flavor with a hint of caramel and a cinnamon-mocha aroma. Use it in pancakes, breads, muffins, cookies and cakes.

Millet flour

This flour has a slightly sweet, cornlike, nutty flavor. It's best used as approximately one-fourth of a flour blend.

Nut flours

Made from ground almonds, chestnuts or hazelnuts, these flours add a rich texture and nutty flavor to baked goods.

Potato flour

This flour has a heavy texture. Use it in small amounts. Potato flour is not the same as potato starch, and the two can't be interchanged.

Potato starch

It works best when it makes up about one-third of a flour blend. Sift or whisk potato starch before adding it to other ingredients to help prevent clumping.

Quinoa flour

With a slightly nutty but strong flavor, quinoa flour can easily overpower baked goods. Limit it to one-fourth of your blend. Try it in highly spiced or flavored foods.

Rice flour (brown)

It is made from whole-grain brown rice and adds a nutty flavor to baked goods. Combine it with other flours and starches. Otherwise, it tends to be gritty, crumbly and dry.

Rice flour (sweet)

This flour is made from sticky short-grain white rice that has more starch than white rice or brown rice. It's also known as sticky, sushi or glutinous rice flour and resembles white rice. It's an excellent thickening agent for sauces, gravies and puddings. It can also be used in small amounts in flour blends.

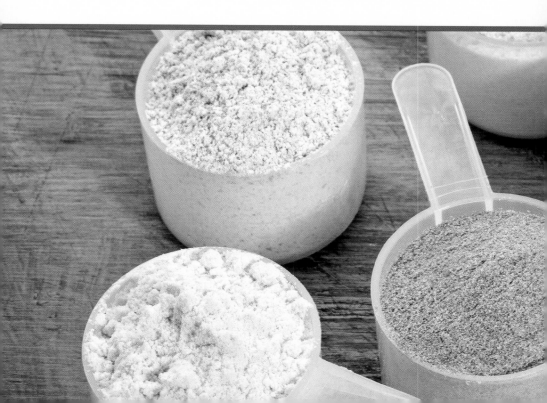

Rice flour (white)

White rice flour is made from ground white rice. This flour has a bland flavor and is best when combined with other gluten-free flours.

Sorghum flour

This is made from ground sorghum (milo). It has a slightly nutty, earthy flavor and works well with bean flours.

Soy flour

Soy flour is made from whole soybeans. It has a strong, nutty flavor. It's best when mixed with other flours and in foods containing nuts, chocolate or spices.

Tapioca flour

This flour can make up about one-fourth to one-half of your flour blend. It can lighten baked goods and create a chewy texture in breads. Use it to thicken soups, gravies, stir-fries and sauces, and as a breading for a crispy coating.

Teff flour

Use this nutty, molasses-like brown flour to make up one-fourth to one-half of a flour blend. It's especially good for dark baked breads, muffins, cookies and cakes. You can also add it to pancakes and puddings. Some teff flour is combined with wheat flour, so buy only 100 percent teff flour.

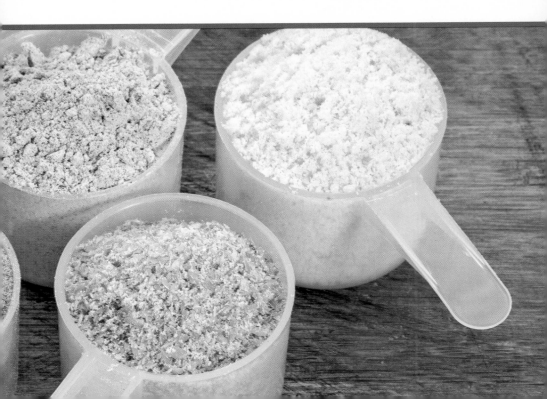

CHAPTER SIXTEEN

Eating away from home

Much of the advice about a gluten-free diet in previous chapters is about cooking and eating in your home. That's as it should be — the foundation of a gluten-free diet lies in your own kitchen. However, a lot of your life takes place outside of your home: at work, at your children's activities, visiting family and friends, on road trips and cross-country flights, at business meetings, and more. A gluten-free diet shouldn't keep you away from any of these events. Plan on being fully engaged in living!

For many people, eating away from home, whether for work or for pleasure, is one of the greatest challenges of a gluten-free diet. You're bound to have some rocky restaurant meals and bumpy travel journeys. When you eat in a cafe or steakhouse, or at a business conference or neighborhood potluck, it's often hard to know if the food you've been served has gluten in it. And it may feel awkward asking about it. Selecting something to eat that you know is safe can be difficult.

But that doesn't mean you can never leave the safety of your own kitchen or that you should eat food that contains gluten to avoid the social awkwardness. As you gain more experience and confidence, you'll find you can eat gluten-free when eating out, and you can enjoy the experience. It all starts with planning and preparation before you leave home. It's also about being vigilant, flexible and creative along the way — there are certain things that you simply can't plan for ahead of time.

Being ready to respond to these unexpected challenges can help you take on any social occasion, business interaction or trip. This chapter will provide you with practical strategies and tested tips to ensure that you can have safe, delicious food to eat anywhere you go.

How to enjoy eating out

When you're eating gluten-free, the rules change between your home environment and the world outside. At home, you're in charge. You know what ingredients go into your food and how they're prepared. And you can always adapt or change recipes, as needed. This level of control typically doesn't exist outside of your home. Restaurants and banquet halls aren't always equipped to prepare gluten-free food. You may not be able to make special dining requests at a social event. When you travel, you may be unfamiliar with stores and restaurants that offer gluten-free foods.

These are some of the common challenges that you may face away from home. For each or these challenges, you can have a response ready to help you overcome it. Don't let food obstacles hold you back from doing the things you want to do. Take a positive, proactive approach. A gluten-free diet may dampen your ability to be spontaneous when eating away from home, but it shouldn't cramp your style.

When eating out, keep in mind that some situations you can change and others you have little influence over. Devote your energy to the things you can change. For example, restaurant dining is something over which you may have some control. You may not be able to change the menu, but with the help of the chef you should be able to find something you can eat. Special events, on the other hand, may operate with a fixed menu. You may not find any food that's gluten-free.

Regardless of your ability to control the situation, approach each occasion with a versatile can-do attitude and a sense of humor. Sometimes, a simple laugh can help you connect with others and diffuse the tension.

The best approach when eating away from home is to plan ahead and be sure you'll always have something safe to eat. This may take some getting used to at first, but soon it will become second nature.

Eating at restaurants

Gluten-free dining has become a hot trend in recent years. Because of this, many restaurants now offer gluten-free meals. This is a good thing for anyone who needs to avoid gluten. But don't forget that restaurants are busy, bustling, boisterous places with a high rate of employee turnover. Even in establishments committed to offering gluten-free options and educating staff about cross-contamination, mistakes can happen. Anytime you eat in a restaurant you need to be very specific about your dining needs.

Also keep in mind that restaurants serve many customers who choose to eat gluten-free, but who don't have to. It's not a medical necessity that they avoid gluten. These individuals may not be as diligent in their efforts to stay away from gluten. They may order a gluten-free meal and top it off with a gluten-containing drink, such as a beer. This can be confusing for restaurant staff and water down the importance of strict gluten avoidance. So don't be surprised if wait staff or kitchen help don't seem as concerned about gluten avoidance or cross-contamination as you might like. Make sure to state that you need to avoid gluten for medical reasons.

CHOOSING A PLACE TO EAT A gluten-free meal starts long before you're seated and you've placed your order. Your first step is choosing a restaurant with gluten-free meal options. Dining in an unknown, out-of-the-way restaurant on the spur of the moment when you're already terribly famished can go terribly awry. It's far better to plan ahead, if possible, so you know you'll have something safe to eat.

You may be able to simply show up and sit down at those restaurants that you know well. But you may need to curb your impromptu approach when dining out in new locations, especially when you travel.

Oftentimes, a fine dining restaurant with a knowledgeable chef is your best bet for enjoying a gluten-free meal. A chain restaurant is also a possibility, since chains often have standardized menus and well-established training programs.

On the other hand, some ethnic restaurants may be a challenge. Traditional Mexican, Asian and Middle Eastern dishes often include sauces and seasonings that contain gluten. Language differences also can make it difficult to communicate your needs. You might consider waiting to visit these types of restaurants until you're more comfortable selecting what to eat, and you're better able to verify that the ingredients are truly gluten-free.

Don't assume that all eateries can accommodate gluten-free requests. If possible, check out the menu online before you go. If you have any questions, call the restaurant during off-peak hours and ask to speak to a manager, owner or chef. Explain that you need to avoid eating gluten. Here are some questions you might ask:

⁎ Do you have gluten-free options?
⁎ Can some menu items be adapted and made gluten-free?
⁎ What precautions do you take to prevent cross-contamination?
⁎ Have members of your staff completed a gluten-free training program?

If a restaurant employee can't answer your questions confidently, consider choosing a different restaurant. Or try booking a table at a less busy time, when servers and chefs aren't rushed and are better able to cater to your needs. Until you're well-versed in gluten-free dining, you might want to bring your dietary guidelines with you in case you need them.

Over time, you'll figure out which restaurants do the best job of preparing delicious gluten-free meals that you enjoy. Consider becoming a regular at

Questions to ask at a restaurant

When selecting a particular menu item, ask your server about the ingredients and preparation methods until you're satisfied that the food is safe for you to eat. Recipes vary from restaurant to restaurant, so always ask how a dish is prepared. Depending on what you order, here's a sampling of questions you might ask to investigate the ingredients in your food:

» What are all the ingredients in this food? (If you simply ask about gluten, you may miss some hidden sources, such as malt vinegar.)
» Is the meat, fish or vegetable seasoned with anything? Has it been marinated in any sauce?
» Do you dust items with flour before sautéing them?
» Do you toast buns or bread on your grill? If so, can you ask the chef to clean the grill before preparing my food?
» Are your French fries or hash browns made from fresh potatoes?
» Are your French fries cooked in a separate fryer from other foods (for example, items coated with breading)?
» Is the bacon included in the meal real or artificial?
» Is the salad topped with croutons or garnished with a bread stick?
» Are any ingredients in your salad dressing made from wheat or barley?
» Do you add wheat to the egg mix used for your omelets?
» Is your rice cooked with bouillon or other seasonings? Is it cooked or warmed in the same water as your pasta?

If you feel embarrassed or intimidated by the idea of playing 20 questions with your server, remember it's very unlikely you're the most demanding customer the restaurant has ever served. Many diners ask a lot of questions and make unconventional requests, even when they don't have a medical condition to look out for! Just remember to be courteous.

these restaurants. Your meals may get better as the restaurant personnel gets to know you.

If you're not in charge of picking the restaurant for a social outing or business dinner, do the best you can to find something on the menu that's safe for you to eat. Pack some snacks just in case that's not possible.

ORDERING YOUR FOOD No restaurant wants you to get a meal that you can't eat — let alone, a meal that can make you sick. Tell your server in a firm yet polite way exactly what you can and can't eat. There are many restaurant employees involved in preparing and serving your meal, and you can't talk to all of them. Ask your server to communicate your needs to anyone who may come in contact with your food.

If you have celiac disease, you may want to tell restaurant staff that you have celiac disease and are allergic to gluten. Celiac disease is an immune response and not an allergic response, but describing your condition in this

Handy cards to have when dining out

It's a good idea to carry gluten-free dining-out cards when you eat out to help communicate your dietary needs. The cards contain a clear written description of the foods and preparation methods that are important in a gluten-free diet. Some free versions of the cards are available on the Web.

You can give a card to your server at any restaurant to explain your needs. Your server can pass it directly to the chef in the kitchen, rather than trying to relay what you just said. This puts a printed description of your dietary needs directly into the hands of the person who's making your food.

A dining-out card doesn't allow you to avoid a candid conversation with your server. You'll still need to ask questions and take sensible precautions. However, a written description in clear language can facilitate better communication and understanding.

Dining-out cards are available in many different languages, so you can take them along if you're traveling abroad. Translated versions often reference foods from a specific region to help you better understand what you can and can't eat. This can be a huge help in arranging safe meals when you're in a foreign country.

way will catch their attention and convey the message that if you eat gluten you'll become ill.

In general, consider ordering the simplest dishes — such as green salads, plain vegetables, and a piece of meat, chicken or fish — especially when you're dining in a restaurant for the first time. Avoid breaded or batter-coated foods, prepared sauces, and gravies, as well as any dish that contains multiple or unfamiliar ingredients, unless you can be assured that they're gluten-free. Beware that many restaurant soups contain flour or a soup base, which contains gluten. Restaurant salad dressings often contain gluten as well. Ask for balsamic or wine vinegar and oil or lemon juice to dress your salad.

If you can't confirm that a food is gluten-free, be prepared to order something else, even if it's not exactly what you want. A safe meal is your highest priority.

If you tend to order the same menu items at the same restaurants, be sure to periodically recheck the ingredients used. Restaurants sometimes change food suppliers, and a new supplier may use different gluten-containing ingredients.

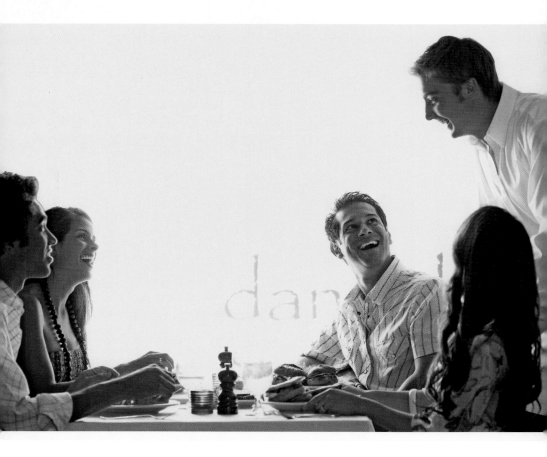

No matter how carefully you order, always inspect your dish for any unpleasant surprises. If you receive a dish with gluten by mistake, don't be afraid to send it back, even if it takes you a few bites to discover the problem.

Don't continue eating something that you believe has gluten in it. Politely explain what needs to be fixed. Let your server know that scraping a problem food off your plate isn't a workable solution — you need a fresh plate that has never had any gluten-containing ingredients on it. Most restaurants are happy to fix a mistake so that you leave as a satisfied customer.

Eating at catered events

Holiday parties, benefits and fundraisers, weddings, banquets, work conferences, and other catered get-togethers can be more intimidating than eating at a restaurant. The food served at these occasions is often a fixed menu — the selections are generally intended for broad appeal, not individual preference. You may not be able to order something different. In addition, you may not have the undivided attention of a server committed to answering your questions in exchange for a generous tip! With practice, you'll learn to navigate these gatherings, so you can confidently celebrate with friends or colleagues.

If you can, find out from the event organizer ahead of time if he or she can prepare a gluten-free meal. It's best to communicate with the catering company directly, if possible. Nowadays, more RSVPs include a gluten-free dining option, right alongside the vegetarian offering, so your needs may be easily accommodated.

During the event, be prepared that the catering staff may not be very familiar with the food they're serving. They may not be able to answer your questions or be able to find someone who can. When in doubt, go without! Eat only the foods that you are certain are gluten-free, and expect to say no to a number of offerings.

In general, fresh fruits and vegetables and cheese plates are usually safe. So are simply prepared vegetables, meat and fish. Don't take a chance on dips, soups or prepared sauces.

The best strategy is to eat something before you go to a catered event so that you're not hungry when you arrive. And make it a habit to take some gluten-free foods with you — such as nuts, dried fruit or gluten-free crackers — in case your options are limited or questionable, or there's a mistake with your meal request.

Also, remember that the food being served is just one of many elements that can make a holiday bash or business event enjoyable. If the gluten-free food options are a bust, concentrate on enjoying the event itself and socializing with those around you.

Eating at other people's homes

There's no reason why you can't say yes to dinner invitations, parties and holiday celebrations that you want to attend. Will your host know what to cook for you or how to avoid gluten cross-contamination? Maybe or maybe not. Concentrate on enjoying the event rather than worrying about the food that you'll be served.

That said, don't be afraid to let people know about your dietary needs in advance. As in a restaurant, politely explain your medical condition and what you can and can't eat, as well as the importance of preventing cross-contamination. Be ready with suggestions that your host might easily prepare. Depending on your relationship with your host, you may offer to bring food to the occasion. If you can supply at least one dish that isn't dessert, you're assured of something you can safely eat at the main meal. Be sure to take your portion from an undisturbed section of the serving dish to avoid cross-contamination.

You may feel sheepish about calling in advance, but remember that it's far less awkward for your host to discover that soy sauce contains gluten before adding it to the entire meal. And it's perfectly acceptable to offer to bring gluten-free bread or to suggest a particular brand of gluten-free ice cream.

At the occasion, do your best to help the evening go as smoothly as possible. There are bound to be a few missteps when people who aren't familiar with the gluten-free diet try to cook for you. When those moments occur, reassure your friends, neighbors and co-workers that their conversation and camaraderie are far more important to you than whatever is being served for dinner. And you can toast your host's willingness to give gluten-free cooking a try!

Eating while traveling

Whether you're traveling for business or for pleasure, a gluten-free diet shouldn't slow you down. Some of the same strategies discussed for eating at local restaurants apply when you travel.

There's a crucial distinction, however, and it's an obvious one. Your ability to make good food choices goes hand in hand with your knowledge of specific ingredients and dishes. If you're not familiar with the local customs, the style of cuisine and the language — in the case of foreign travel — eating gluten-free can be more difficult.

Does that mean you should ditch your vacation plans and stick only to places you're familiar with? Absolutely not! Some basic strategies can help in avoiding gluten. Be prepared that you may need to work a little bit more and plan ahead more than normal.

If you're just getting used to a gluten-free diet, short stints to big cities are a good way to start. Big cities offer more eating variety and restaurants are used to special orders. Once you're comfortable eating gluten-free food on the go, you can confidently hop a plane, train or automobile to any location you like.

BEFORE YOU GO When doing your research, determine which airlines, hotels, resorts, bed-and-breakfasts, tour groups, or cruise lines are good at catering to your dietary needs. There are several websites and travel agencies that can help you do this.

Sampling the local cuisine is part of the adventure when you travel. If possible, make arrangements that allow you to eat gluten-free versions of the local fare rather than eating a bland chicken breast every night. To make things easier, there are tours and cruises available — even gluten-free travel clubs — specifically designed for individuals who need to avoid gluten.

Also consider a hotel room or condo that includes a kitchen or kitchenette, so you can prepare some of your own meals. Or you can request a small

Visiting other countries

If you travel abroad, be aware that the level of awareness about gluten will vary from region to region and country to country. Do your research and make sure you're up for the challenge before you book the trip. You might begin by visiting the websites of travel agencies that cater to individuals with special dietary needs.

If you're struggling with the details, seek out personal experiences shared by other travelers. Online celiac disease support groups often share inside tips and advice that can make your travel experience more enjoyable. Celiac disease support groups in the regions where you'll be traveling are also excellent sources of local tourist information.

Wherever you go, careful planning and extra effort upfront are difference-makers. You don't have to plan every meal in advance, but it's important to be prepared and informed. Pack food and snacks, as needed. That way, you're less likely to get sick, hungry or forced into eating something you're not sure about. It's also wise to take along gluten-free dining-out cards in the native language of each of the countries you're visiting (see page 236). They may save a lot of time and frustration in finding gluten-free meals.

Your goal is to enjoy the experience and the sights, not worry about finding something to eat!

Tasty travel snacks

Here are some options for gluten-free snacks to take with you when traveling:

- Rice cakes
- Fresh fruit and vegetables
- Dried fruit
- Nuts
- Trail mix

- Gluten-free crackers or chips
- Gluten-free cookies
- Gluten-free protein or energy bars
- Corn chips
- Popcorn

If you can, pack a container of gluten-free peanut butter or hummus for dipping. If you have a cooler or ice pack, you could include yogurt, cheese sticks, or sandwiches or wraps prepared at home.

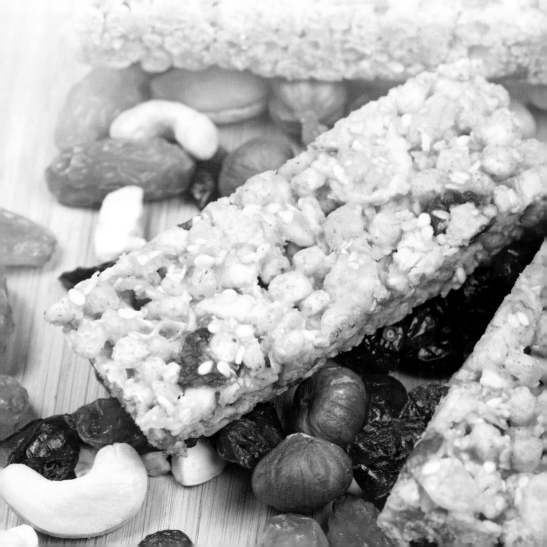

refrigerator or microwave be placed in your room for medical reasons. Make sure the kitchens are clean, and take precautions to avoid cross-contamination.

When you arrive at your destination, hotel staff or your tour guide may be able to identify restaurants and stores nearby that offer gluten-free options, but it's good to be aware of some resources in advance.

Last but not least, pack your bags with your gluten-free diet in mind. Depending on your travel plans, you may want to pack gluten-free bread, snacks or other hard-to-find items in your luggage. It's also wise to take along gluten-free dining-out cards.

EN ROUTE If you're taking a road trip, pack a cooler full of healthy gluten-free snacks and beverages, since many fast food restaurants and truck stops have limited gluten-free options. If you're flying or traveling by bus or train, pack enough food to carry you through the trip in case there's a mistake with your gluten-free meal or you can't find good gluten-free options along the way. Plan for layovers and delays. Just make sure you understand restrictions or requirements about what you may carry with you as you pass through security checks.

If you requested gluten-free travel meals in advance, double-check with staff that the meals don't contain gluten. Don't assume anything. When the meal arrives, inspect its contents. If you have any doubt about the ingredients, opt for the snacks you packed instead.

AT YOUR DESTINATION As much as possible, stick to your typical eating routine when you travel. Check menus online or with a phone app, or you can stop by a restaurant during slower times to discuss your dietary needs. Purchase naturally gluten-free foods from grocery stores and kiosks to have available as a backup. Make sure to read food labels to verify the ingredients.

If you're traveling in a foreign country and you don't speak the language fluently, consider enlisting the help of the staff and concierge at your hotel to communicate your dietary needs. They may be able to help book a restaurant reservation for you and alert the restaurant staff about your dietary restrictions. Or they may be able to help arrange tours and sightseeing trips that can accommodate special meal requests.

Finally, beware that gluten-free labeling laws vary from country to country. If you plan to grocery shop on your trip outside the United States, spend time beforehand learning about the cuisine and the common ingredients and seasonings of the countries you're visiting. If possible, learn to recognize food names in the native language.

Cheers!

Whether you're toasting in a local banquet hall, a friend's home or a French bistro, you can celebrate in style and still stay committed to your gluten-free diet. You can also enjoy an alcoholic beverage, as long as you choose wisely (see page 169).

As you've learned in this chapter, your success depends on your ability to plan ahead, to communicate your dietary needs clearly, and to manage mistakes and mishaps. Keeping a package of nuts in your pocket at all times doesn't hurt either!

CHAPTER SEVENTEEN

Handling the bumps

Like many people learning to live with a gluten- or wheat-related disorder, you may be struggling with a mixture of emotions, everything from anger and denial to relief and, finally, acceptance. Understanding the reasons behind your symptoms has likely taken a weight off your shoulders. At the same time, discovering that you have an illness that you'll have to deal with the rest of your life can be overwhelming. You may find yourself wondering if life will ever be normal again.

Having celiac disease or being sensitive to gluten or wheat can be stressful and isolating at times, particularly because the burden of successful treatment rests squarely with you. There's no surgery or pill that can fix your problem. It's all about carefully managing your diet. Take comfort in knowing that people who begin to follow a gluten-free diet often experience significant improvements in their quality of life within the first year, and often in the first few months.

As you may be discovering, though, going gluten-free involves more than what you put in your mouth. Managing life on a gluten-free diet can affect your social life and emotions in ways you may not have anticipated. The first six months tend to be especially challenging. Hang in there. With time, the change in your lifestyle often becomes second nature. By choosing to be proactive rather than reactive, your condition won't control you. You can learn to control it.

Adapting to change

Life is full of change. Some changes are anticipated and happy, such as finding a loving life companion or a fulfilling job. Others are more difficult — losing a loved one or going through a divorce. Difficult life changes can be overwhelming, and experiencing a chronic illness is no different.

Getting diagnosed with celiac disease involves two major life changes: learning to with live with a chronic illness and starting on a lifelong gluten-free diet. If you experienced severe symptoms, the relief that comes with a diagnosis may make the adjustment easier. In comparison, if you experienced mild or "silent" symptoms, the adjustment may be more challenging because the benefits of a gluten-free diet aren't as obvious. If you have non-celiac gluten sensitivity, depending on your circumstances, you may also experience significant change.

During this period of adjustment, you may experience some form of loss. It's important to acknowledge and grieve that loss, no matter how great or small. You may also begin to feel anxious, uneasy and vulnerable. You may even feel that your body has turned against you and that you've lost control over your life. These feelings can lead to anxiety about how you'll cope with the requirements of a gluten-free diet. After a while, though, as you become more familiar with your new way of life, you'll notice that you're gaining more confidence, and you're more optimistic about your ability to enjoy life without gluten. You may even begin looking forward to the possibilities that lie before you.

IT'S ALL ABOUT ATTITUDE The way you handle this major change in your life is perhaps the most influential factor in determining its impact on your health and happiness. Your attitude, along with your social and spiritual ties, are tools you can use to more successfully adjust to change, no matter where life's path may take you. You'll find that an optimistic attitude can make your days more enjoyable and less stressful.

In general, optimists are convinced they can change and make things work out. They tend to react to difficult situations by taking action. Negative or pessimistic thoughts, on the other hand, can intensify stress and frustration. People generally don't choose to be optimists or pessimists. The attitude you take toward life events is likely a combination of genetics, early environment and life experiences. But that doesn't mean you're stuck with your attitude. Pessimism can be changed to some degree. By being mindful of the ways in which your viewpoint brings you down or influences how you think, you may be able to approach certain events in a different manner.

Pay attention to the messages you constantly give yourself. When you catch yourself thinking that life is terrible, stop the thought in its tracks.

If the changes your illness has brought to your life have you struggling to keep a smile on your face, experiment with the following suggestions to see if they can help you:

- **Do things you enjoy.** You may be inclined to give up enjoyable activities and avoid responsibility. This type of withdrawal from life can make you feel worse and cause you to feel stuck.
- **Take care of yourself.** That means eating right, exercising regularly, making sleep a priority, and avoiding drugs and excessive alcohol.
- **Look for fun forms of exercise.** Regular exercise can improve your mood and increase your sense of confidence and well-being. It can serve as a distraction from negative thoughts, and it can open up opportunities to socialize.
- **Talk to someone.** Don't hide your struggles from those who are close to you. Share your problems with a trusted friend or a family member. Or seek out the camaraderie of a support group in your area. The important thing is to stay connected.
- **Avoid negative people.** The better you feel emotionally, the better able you'll be physically and mentally to cope with your diet change. Cultivate relationships with people who boost you up rather than bring you down.
- **Use distraction.** Take a walk or engage in a hobby to refocus your mind away from worries or negative thoughts.
- **Maintain a regular schedule.** As much as possible, stick to a varied and regular routine that includes hobbies as well as work. Having a predictable schedule will create a sense of stability and control in the face of your illness.
- **Enjoy a good laugh.** Not everything has to be deep and dark. Laughter relieves tension and relaxes your muscles as well as your mind. Lighten up with a funny movie. Spend time with people who take themselves lightly or have a sense of humor.

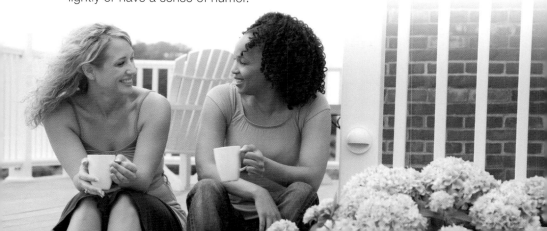

Instead, make a mental list of all the things you take for granted but for which you are truly grateful.

How you experience life without gluten will depend in large part on the attitude you take. It's OK, necessary even, to give yourself space to grieve. In time, though, you'll be able to turn the page on one chapter of life and move on to the next. Moving forward with acceptance and a positive outlook will allow you to embrace your new life rather than feel burdened by it.

Caring for your overall health

As you work to adopt a gluten-free lifestyle you'll no doubt encounter bumps along the way. Among other things, you may find that a complete change in what you eat doesn't alleviate all of the physical and mental challenges associated with needing to avoid gluten. You may be struggling with problems such as anxiety, depression, constipation or irritable bowel syndrome. These difficulties can affect your desire to interact with the world around you, but with some active problem-solving, you can address many of the issues that may be interfering with your enjoyment of life.

DEPRESSION AND ANXIETY Before you realized that your body couldn't tolerate gluten, your symptoms may have taken a physical and emotional toll that left you feeling depleted and emotionally drained. Now you may feel out of sorts for different reasons. Going gluten-free takes time and energy, and it can lead to feelings of isolation, frustration and stress. The fear of inadvertently exposing yourself to gluten may cause you to worry more than you'd like. You may also feel discouraged and pessimistic about the future.

Know that you're not alone. People with celiac disease seem to be more likely to suffer from depression and anxiety than the general population. Research also shows that women tend to be more affected than men. As with many chronic conditions, give it time. Research shows depression and quality of life improve when people with celiac disease stick to a gluten-free diet.

It's also worth noting that the link between celiac disease and depression may be more complex than just the physical and emotional strain of living with a chronic illness. Other conditions associated with celiac disease, such as thyroid disease, are known to cause depression. It's also possible that certain nutritional deficiencies related to the disease may play a role. Seeking the help of a medical professional can have a positive effect.

Regardless of the cause, understanding depression and anxiety, and learning positive ways to respond to it, can make a big difference in your health and well-being.

Understanding depression and anxiety Everyone feels blue now and then. Depression is different. It's a serious health problem — not a passing phase that goes away on its own. It can cause general feelings of unhappiness and hopelessness, as well as physical symptoms such as headaches, bellyaches or back pain. Weight changes and sleep problems also are common signs and symptoms of depression. So are fatigue, difficulty concentrating and a lack of enjoyment in pleasurable activities. Research has shown that depression can affect your ability to adhere to a gluten-free diet, which can make you feel worse.

Anxiety often accompanies depression, and it usually involves excessive, irrational fear and dread. Symptoms can include muscle tension, body aches, sweating, and feeling scared, restless or on edge. Anxiety can also cause irritability, sleep problems, fatigue and difficulty concentrating.

As with depression, high levels of anxiety can negatively affect your mood, relationships and enjoyment of life. Anxiety also makes performing tasks and coping with a chronic illness more difficult.

If you think you may be experiencing symptoms of depression, anxiety or both, talk to your doctor. Eliminating depression and anxiety can help you better cope with your condition and improve your overall quality of life.

BATHROOM WOES When you went on a gluten-free diet, you expected all of your gastrointestinal troubles to go away, but they haven't. In addition to celiac disease, some people also experience irritable bowel syndrome (IBS) or lactose intolerance. Despite getting rid of gluten, they continue to experience abdominal pain or discomfort, bloating, and diarrhea.

Constipation also can be a problem. Constipation may occur with IBS. It can also result from a change in diet. When you eliminate gluten, you're more likely to eat foods lower in fiber. Too little fiber can lead to constipation. A diet that includes gluten-free foods higher in fiber will help treat constipation.

It can be frustrating when gastrointestinal symptoms persist, and it may take a bit of time for you and your doctor to determine what's going on and how to solve the problem. But just because your gut is somewhat unpredictable, don't let that keep you from doing things outside the home.

These tips can reduce the stress and worry of your gut flaring up in public:

❋ **Travel wisely.** If you're walking to your destination, consider planning your route ahead of time to get to where you're going as quickly as possible. If you are making a long drive, know the distance between restrooms on your route. When traveling by plane, ask to sit in an aisle seat that's close to the restroom. You can also take advantage of websites and apps that help you locate nearby restrooms worldwide.

- **Carry a survival kit.** You'll be more likely to enjoy yourself if you feel secure. Some people find it helpful to bring a change of clothes and a small emergency supply of tissue when they are out and about. You might also include medication to treat diarrhea or constipation.

- **Get your bearings in new places.** When going to a new restaurant, home or other location, find out where the restrooms are. At restaurants, ask to sit near the restroom if possible.

- **Try to relax.** Stress can cause your symptoms to act up. If you feel a little nervous before going to a party or social occasion, practice relaxation exercises such as meditation, muscle relaxation or relaxed breathing.

Coping with social issues

For better or worse, socializing with friends and family often involves eating. The sharing of food is a common way that people come together. Food symbolizes similarities rather than differences. Now that you need to avoid gluten, you're finding that socializing is more complicated — even stressful. You may find yourself avoiding social occasions for fear of eating the wrong foods, feeling deprived and left out, or being a burden to the hostess.

It's normal to experience some worry or social anxiety when it comes to eating away from home. It can be uncomfortable and isolating to watch friends, family or co-workers enjoying food while you abstain. You may feel ignored or invisible. On the other hand, you may feel that people are staring at you, wondering why you aren't eating along with everyone else. You may feel like you're in the spotlight and you don't fit in. With practice and patience, you can learn to handle these social hurdles with self-confidence and poise. Being on a gluten-free diet shouldn't dictate your social life or interfere with being able to have fun with others (see Chapter 16).

DEALING WITH FEELINGS OF ISOLATION Just because you're on a gluten-free diet doesn't mean that you can't engage in the same activities you always have. In fact, it's important that you socialize and stay active. Whereas social isolation can contribute to illness and poor health, strong family ties and good friendships contribute to mental and emotional well-being.

If being on a gluten-free diet is causing you to feel isolated, consider the following suggestions:

- **Speak up for yourself.** At first you may feel awkward or embarrassed when requesting a gluten-free meal at a restaurant or social occasion.

There's nothing to be embarrassed about. The awkwardness you feel will diminish or disappear over time.

🌸 **Be open with those you trust.** People will be better able to support you if you take the time to educate them about your illness. Keeping the lines of communication open is good. You'll feel less isolated and more connected.

🌸 **Be the host.** Many people on a gluten-free diet find eating at home less troublesome than eating out. If that's the case for you, consider hosting more social gatherings in your home. Prepare a festive gluten-free meal to share.

🌸 **Suggest a restaurant.** If you don't want to cook, bring people together at a restaurant that you've come to know and trust.

🌸 **Take control.** Feeling secure in a social setting will enable you to better enjoy yourself. Do what you need to do to feel comfortable. If you're going to a social event, call ahead of time to find out what's being served and politely explain your dietary needs. Offer to bring a dish or two to share.

🌸 **Make relationships a priority.** Healthy, fulfilling long-term relationships are important. Don't take your spouse, partner, family or friends for granted. Make time to regularly do something with those who are important to you.

INTERACTING WITH OTHERS One of the biggest dilemmas you may face is when — and how — to tell others about your disease or condition. In some cases, you may prefer to avoid bringing up the topic, but you're likely to encounter situations in which addressing your condition is a necessity. For example, if you'll be attending a dinner, it's best to call ahead to explain your situation and find out what food will be served. When eating with a new friend or acquaintance, it's likely the subject may come up. One option is to address it at the start of the meal so that you can put it aside and move on to other conversational topics. Another option is not to bring up the topic unless your friend inquires.

Depending on the circumstances and the person involved, you may choose to give a brief or a more detailed explanation of your disorder. You may simply say that your body cannot tolerate gluten. Or you may explain that you have a condition that requires you to avoid all foods that contain gluten. If you

Maintaining a lifelong gluten-free diet is the only treatment for celiac disease. Research shows that anywhere from 36 to 90 percent of people with celiac disease adhere to a strict gluten-free diet. If you experienced severe symptoms before learning of your disease, your motivation to avoid gluten may be quite strong. If, on the other hand, your symptoms were mild or you didn't have any symptoms, you may find going gluten-free to be more of a challenge.

Regardless of your circumstances, you'll likely face moments of temptation. Perhaps you suddenly crave pizza from your local pizzeria. Or you experience the urge to indulge in a favorite dessert at a party. You may also be tempted to eat unsafe foods simply to please others. You fear that you'll offend a friend if you turn down that casserole she's so carefully prepared. Or while at a restaurant with business associates, instead of going through the hassle and embarrassment of returning a meal that's been contaminated with gluten, you simply eat it.

If you're having difficulty adhering to a gluten-free diet and you're tempted to cheat, here are some tips to try:

> **Focus on what you can eat.** Instead of thinking about what you can't eat, think about the wide variety of foods that you can eat. Savor the gluten-free foods you enjoy.
> **Eat before going out.** If you think you'll be tempted by food offered at a party or social gathering, eat something beforehand so that you aren't hungry when you arrive. It's easier to resist temptation when you're not hungry.
> **Reward yourself.** When you do resist temptation, reward yourself with something you enjoy, such as a manicure or a round of golf.

How to respond when you feel the urge to cheat

have celiac disease, you might want to mention that eating gluten can cause permanent damage to your body. There are a variety of responses you can give — short and sweet or more detailed — depending on who's inquiring.

Don't be surprised if you encounter some people who don't seem to comprehend your condition. Perhaps a friend serves breaded chicken and a salad with croutons, despite knowing about your dietary needs. She thinks you just can't eat bread or pasta. Or a relative urges you to "just have a taste" of his daughter's wedding cake. Try to keep in mind that most of the time, people are well-meaning. They simply don't understand that even a small amount of gluten can wreak havoc on your body. Remember, neither did you before your diagnosis! Give them some slack. Rather than assuming these individuals are willfully ignoring your needs or intentionally leaving you out, take the time to politely explain your situation.

Even after you take the time to educate people about your condition, some still may not understand the importance of a gluten-free diet. They may think you're overreacting or being picky, or that a little gluten is OK. If you're encountering this kind of resistance, you might consider offering a book or website that explains your disorder. Or invite them to come with you to an appointment with your doctor or dietitian. If all else fails, you may have to accept that some people just aren't capable of changing their mindset. It's OK to protect yourself from negative or critical people, but don't let one person cause you to miss out on an opportunity to socialize with others. Try to maintain a positive outlook.

Functioning well as a family

Like you, it may take your family time to adjust to your new diet. They're coming to terms with what it means to live with someone who needs to adhere to a strict diet. They may be worried about your health and wonder how to help you manage your diet. Or they may worry that now they'll have to eat the same things you do. They may also be frustrated that you can no longer go to some of their favorite restaurants because you can't eat the food there. Celiac disease and related disorders are a family affair, like it or not. But be patient. Management of your condition represents a major life change for your family and, just as you will, they'll need time to adapt.

HOW YOU CAN HELP YOUR FAMILY Some families rally quickly, offering full support. Others don't. Some people confront resistance or frustration from their closest family members. Your spouse may resent the additional time and money spent on maintaining a gluten-free diet. Your children may not understand the importance of cleaning up crumbs or thoroughly washing utensils. They may miss the spontaneity of ordering out for pizza, stopping for fast food or dropping in at a friend's house for lunch. They may feel that your needs have taken precedence over theirs.

With some understanding and effort on your part, your family can over-come many of their frustrations and concerns. Here are some tips to help them along the way:

- **Educate them.** Your family needs to understand how gluten affects your body and why you need to avoid it. If possible, bring them to your appointments with your dietitian or doctor. Encourage them to attend support group meetings. The more they know, the more they'll be able to support you with understanding and compassion.

- **Help them let go of guilt.** It's not unusual for family members to experience guilt when indulging in "forbidden" foods in your presence. It can take away from the pleasure and fun of attending social events. Let them know it's OK to enjoy the foods they love.

- **Agree on a meal plan.** Some families choose to eat gluten-free meals together. Others prefer to eat separate meals. Or you can combine both options. Perhaps you share gluten-free dinners but prepare separate meals for breakfast and lunch. Whatever you choose, make sure it's something you decide on together.

- **Improvise on holiday traditions.** At yearly gatherings, both you and your family may find it distressing that some foods may be off-limits. Be creative. Try making gluten-free stuffing to share on Thanksgiving or gluten-free cake on birthdays. Many traditional meals can be modified — de-glutenized — without affecting their quality.

- **Balance your needs with theirs.** It's important that you create a safe eating environment at home and when you're out and about. On the other hand, don't let your gluten-free diet become the primary focus of family life. On occasion, go to a restaurant your family enjoys, even though it may not suit your needs (and bring a snack that you can eat). Let your family know that you don't mind doing this because you know they make sacrifices for you.

- **Keep the lines of communication open.** Talk about any concerns you have and give your family members the chance to do the same. Keep an open mind. Be willing to problem-solve together when difficulties or frustrations arise.

HOW YOUR FAMILY CAN HELP YOU Your family also may be struggling with how to best support you. Here are some suggestions for them to consider:

- **Don't second-guess.** You, more than anyone, understand your body and your illness. Your family should avoid second-guessing you. By trusting you and supporting your choices, they'll increase your confidence in your ability to handle your condition.

❋ **Be supportive but not overprotective.** It's one thing for your family to offer support. It's another to constantly ask if you're OK or if you need something — or worse, if you should be eating that. This kind of over-protectiveness can make you feel more, not less, anxious.

❋ **Avoid blame.** Family members may knowingly or unknowingly blame you for the way your condition has changed their lives. It's best if they can acknowledge those feelings and work toward letting go of them.

Dealing with religious matters

It's not something most people think about, but another area that can be a stumbling block for individuals with celiac disease or a related disorder has to do with religion. Because you can't eat gluten, you may not be able to adhere to certain religious practices. Why? The food involved in certain religious traditions is made from wheat. Fortunately, most religions have made adaptations to include individuals on a gluten-free diet.

COMMUNION WAFERS Receiving communion is a meaningful aspect of many Christian religious services. Many churches, including Protestant, Eastern Orthodox, Ancient Eastern and nondenominational, have no specific or written requirements for the grain used to produce a communion wafer. To accommodate people with gluten intolerance, they offer gluten-free communion wafers made of rice- or potato-based flours. Another option is to provide gluten-free bread or crackers.

The Roman Catholic Church has more strict requirements when it comes to communion wafers. According to long-standing teachings, a host can only be consecrated if it's made of wheat and water. Hosts that are completely gluten-free are considered invalid. To accommodate people who cannot consume gluten, the United States Conference of Catholic Bishops has worked with three U.S. distributors of communion wafers to produce extremely low-gluten hosts. If your church doesn't offer this type of wafer, talk to your clergy about obtaining some. If you're extremely sensitive to gluten and your doctor has determined that even a very low-gluten host is unsafe for you, the Catholic Church has indicated that in specific situations Holy Communion may be received under the species of wine only.

Generally, you can drink wine, but it's important that the wine be in a separate glass to avoid contamination. It's best not to drink from a communal chalice. If you must do so, try to be the first person to drink from the chalice. When drinking from a communal chalice, there's a very low risk of cross-contamination if people dip regular wafers that contain gluten in the communal cup.

JEWISH TRADITIONS Consuming certain foods that traditionally contain gluten — namely challah and matzo — is an integral part of the Jewish observance. Jewish law requires that these items be made of one of five grains: wheat, barley, spelt, rye or oats. Since the first four grains contain gluten, challah or matzo made from gluten-free oats is the only acceptable option.

Oat-based challah can be prepared or purchased for religious observances such as Shabbat, the Jewish Sabbath, or Sukkoth, the harvest holiday. If you don't have access to gluten-free challah, or if your doctor has determined that you shouldn't eat gluten-free oats, Jewish teaching states that it's acceptable to bypass the ritual of eating challah.

Pesach, also known as Passover, presents additional concerns if you need to avoid gluten. One of the primary religious requirements at the Passover Seder meal is to eat matzo. Matzo is traditionally made from wheat flour, but several U.S. distributors make oat-based matzo that's kosher for Passover. Whether oat-based matzo is an acceptable substitute at the Seder depends on which traditions you follow. You may want to consult your rabbi for clarification. Your rabbi may also waive the requirement to consume matzo at the Seder meal if your doctor has determined that oat-based matzo isn't a safe option for you.

Enjoying a full life

Living with celiac disease or gluten or wheat sensitivity will undoubtedly present you with other unique challenges. The key is to be patient and give yourself time to adjust to the changes that these challenges represent. Work on accepting the obstacles, and actively seek out solutions. You want to embrace this major life transition with courage and confidence. By understanding situations you may encounter and how to react to them, you'll be better equipped to maintain a gluten-free diet while continuing to engage in a satisfying lifestyle.

CHAPTER EIGHTEEN

Helping your child eat gluten-free

Your daughter is invited to a birthday party where her friends will celebrate with cake. Or your son wants to hang out with "the guys," which usually involves ordering pizza. Situations like these can be challenging for your child if he or she can't eat gluten, and they can be overwhelming for you. After all, you're the one responsible for teaching your child what's safe and unsafe to eat and how to navigate difficult circumstances.

If your child has recently started a gluten-free diet, the sense of responsibility may weigh heavily on you. Along with adjusting to the ins and outs of your child's new diet, you're likely worrying about how it will affect his or her social life and emotional well-being. Will your child feel left out, different or deprived?

It may be comforting to know that parents tend to overestimate the negative effects of the gluten-free diet on their children. If your child is young — under the age of 5 — when you find out that he or she can't eat gluten, chances are the adjustment will be relatively smooth. He or she will soon forget what gluten-containing foods taste like and likely won't miss them. Eating gluten-free will feel normal because it's what your child has always known.

If it's later in childhood or during the teen years that your son or daughter must learn a new diet, the adjustment may be more challenging. Even so, your child will adapt. In fact, research indicates that adults who began eliminating gluten in childhood or adolescence found a gluten-free diet easier to manage than adults who were diagnosed later in life. Adults who are diagnosed as children or teenagers are also more likely to experience a quality of life similar to that of adults who don't have celiac disease.

To be sure, going gluten-free will present your child with some unique challenges. With your guidance, those challenges can be met with increasing confidence and ease. It's a matter of practice, patience and perseverance. In time, you'll notice that your fears about your child's illness lessen considerably. Eventually, maintaining a gluten-free diet will become second nature for both of you.

Important life lessons

One of the greatest gifts you can give your child is a solid understanding of his or her illness and why it's critical to follow a gluten-free diet. Children who are fully educated about their condition and the reasons behind the gluten-free diet are more likely to avoid eating gluten. The opposite is true if they have an incorrect or incomplete understanding of the short- and long-term health effects of consuming gluten.

Educating your child will not only involve ongoing conversations about his or her disorder and foods that are gluten-free. It will also require a gradual shift of responsibility for the diet from you to your child. The idea of giving up even a little control over food choices may seem scary at first, but it's the best way for your child to learn while you're still there to offer guidance.

As your child's knowledge and maturity increases, it's a good idea to gradually extend more trust and control. The ultimate goal is for your youngster to become an independent and self-sufficient adult who is fully invested in staying healthy and adept at doing so. The more opportunities you give your child to learn about and take responsibility for a gluten-free diet, the more confident and capable your child will become.

It's never too early to start the process of educating. Here are some suggestions to increase your child's knowledge and sense of responsibility:

❋ **Encourage active participation at appointments.** Encourage your child to ask questions at doctor and dietitian appointments, and make sure he or she is listening to all that's being said. Let your son or daughter know it's OK to ask questions if something is unclear or doesn't make sense.

- **Teach your child to read food labels.** Being able to determine which foods contain gluten is crucial to successfully maintaining a gluten-free diet. Give your child the tools to decode food labels. If your child can't read yet, take time to read labels aloud.

- **Take your child grocery shopping.** Let him or her help choose which foods to buy for your household. Praise good food choices and explain why other foods aren't safe.

- **Involve your child in meal preparation.** Pass along the skills he or she will need to prepare gluten-free snacks and meals. Ask your child to help pack school lunches.

- **Empower your child to make food choices outside the home.** When eating in restaurants or at social occasions, ask your son or daughter what he or she thinks is safe to eat. If your child points to something containing gluten, use it as an opportunity to educate.

- **See mistakes as opportunities.** There will be times when your child accidentally or purposefully eats food containing gluten. Rather than respond with anger or frustration, try to turn the mistake into a teachable moment. Ask why the choice was made and help your child understand why it wasn't a good one. Remember, making mistakes is part of any learning process.

Helping your child be a child

As your child adjusts to life without gluten, one of the ways you can offer support is by setting up a safe and positive environment at home. More daunting is the prospect of sending your child off into the world, where you can't control everything that enters his or her mouth or how people will respond to his or her condition. You may be concerned about letting your child attend birthday parties, sleepovers or other social occasions.

Your protective instinct is understandable, but it shouldn't prevent your child from leading a full and rich life. Children need the opportunity to negotiate the challenges of life on their own. Having that freedom allows them to develop the skills they will need to be successful and happy adults.

FEARS OF NOT FITTING IN There's nothing more important to a child than fitting in. At times, though, a gluten-free diet may make your child feel different around other kids. Don't shy away from acknowledging this reality.

A number of recent and ongoing medical studies are attempting to determine whether it's possible to lower a child's risk of developing celiac disease. Some studies have looked at the role of breast-feeding. Early results seemed to suggest that breast-feeding may have a protective effect. If you're breast-feeding when you first introduce foods containing gluten into your baby's diet, you might reduce your child's risk of developing celiac disease. Other research raised the idea that the longer you breast-fed, the lower your child's risk of developing celiac disease. More recent studies, however, suggest that breast-feeding may not be a key factor.

The age at which you introduce your infant to gluten-containing foods is being explored as another possible factor in reducing the risk of developing celiac disease. Studies indicate that the ideal time to begin feeding your baby wheat cereal or other gluten-containing foods is between the ages of 4 months and 6 months. Introducing gluten to your baby before or after that window of time may increase his or her chances of developing celiac disease. Starting out with small amounts of food that contain gluten and gradually increasing that amount also may be beneficial. Again, more research is needed to confirm or refute these initial findings.

If celiac disease runs in your family, talk to your doctor about how to best protect your child.

Is it possible to prevent celiac disease in children?

Instead, let your child know that, in a way, being different is actually quite normal. Everyone is different in one way or another and everyone sometimes feels like they don't fit in. Reinforce the idea that your child shouldn't feel ashamed of having to be on a special diet. Encourage him or her to be matter-of-fact in talking about his or her condition to peers and adults. The more open your son or daughter is, the less of an issue it will be and the more comfortable he or she will feel.

Another way to help your child feel more at ease with a gluten-free lifestyle is to seek out support groups. A number of national organizations support kids with gluten disorders, including R.O.C.K. (Raising Our Celiac Kids) and the Cel-Kids Network. Find out if a local support group exists in your area. If not, consider starting one. Your child is likely to benefit significantly from

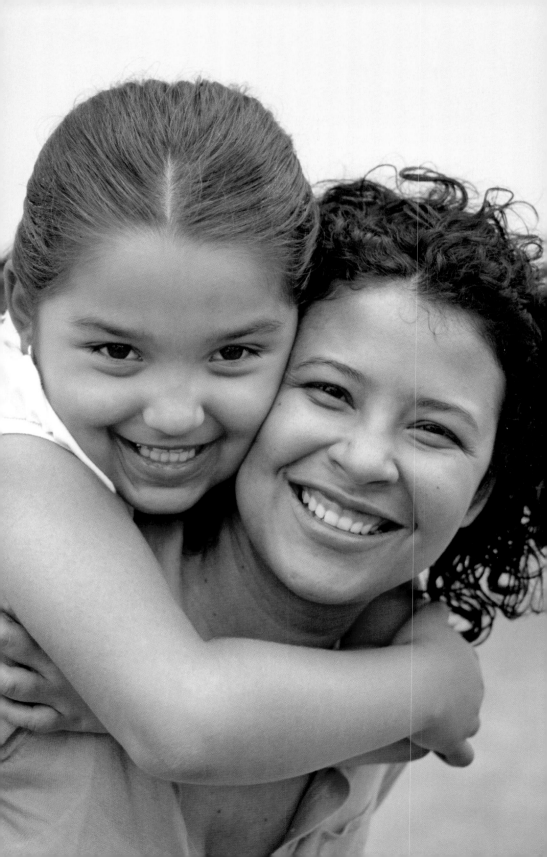

talking to peers who understand exactly what it means to be on a gluten-free diet. Another option to consider is enrolling your child in one of several camps created specifically for kids who can't eat gluten.

Even with your support and guidance, there may be times when your child expresses anger, sadness or frustration. Listen with sympathy and validate those feelings, then encourage your child to focus on the positive. Do your best to model an optimistic attitude. Whether you realize it or not, your child is constantly observing your reactions and following your lead. That includes how you talk about the illness to your child and how you discuss it with others. For suggestions about how to help nurture a positive outlook, turn to Chapter 17.

LIFE OUTSIDE THE HOME The best way to help your child fit in and feel comfortable around other kids is to anticipate difficulties ahead of time. The more prepared you and your child are for food-related issues, the more likely your child will be able to eat safely while still having a good time. To help your child manage social situations, consider these suggestions:

Role play Give your child opportunities to practice speaking up for him- or herself. Pretend you're a friend, family member or other adult. Play out a range of situations and help your child come up with the right language to explain why he or she can't eat something.

Call ahead Whether it's a birthday party at a friend's house or a postgame meal at a restaurant, contact the adult in charge in advance. Explain your child's food restrictions and ask what food will be served. If needed, let the person know that your child will be bringing a gluten-free alternative to eat. As your child gets older, encourage him or her to take on this responsibility.

Always provide safe food alternatives If you know that cake or pizza will be served at a party, be sure to provide a favorite gluten-free alternative for your child. Your child is less likely to feel deprived if a similar or more desirable option is available.

Teach your child to say 'no thank you' Certain well-meaning children or adults may not fully understand your child's need to avoid all gluten. When your child is offered unsafe food, it's important to know how to politely but firmly turn it down.

Set up a trading system at home for forbidden treats Events and holidays such as Halloween can be difficult when your child can't eat gluten. If your child brings home forbidden goodies, consider having a basket full of safe

Celiac disease and type 1 diabetes

It's not uncommon for a child to have both celiac disease and type 1 diabetes. They are both autoimmune diseases with many common genes. By some estimates, up to 10 percent of children with type 1 diabetes also have celiac disease. This is why it's a good idea that a child diagnosed with type 1 diabetes also to be tested for celiac disease, and vice versa. In most children, diabetes is diagnosed before celiac disease, generally because it's more common and because doctors are more familiar with diabetes.

If your child has both conditions, he or she will have to follow a diet that accommodates for both gluten and carbohydrates, which can be challenging. Early on — because the body isn't absorbing food as it should due to celiac disease — monitoring blood sugar levels and determining how much insulin to take can be difficult because of fluctuations in sugar levels. This can lead to episodes of low blood sugar (hypoglycemia). However, as celiac disease and nutrient absorption improve, the process often gets easier.

Expect the amount of insulin your child needs to change as celiac disease improves. Once a child with both conditions is on a gluten-free diet, episodes of hypoglycemia are generally reduced, but it can take several months before the effects become noticeable.

alternatives. That way, your child can trade in an unsafe treat for an equally desirable gluten-free one.

Be prepared for postgame snacks Many kids' sports teams share a snack or celebratory meal after practices and games. Be sure to inform your child's coach about your child's condition. You may also choose to inform other parents if they're taking turns bringing snacks. Just to be safe, make sure your child always packs a favorite gluten-free snack in case others bring something he or she can't eat. And have a plan if your child will be eating out.

Plan ahead for camp Call your child's camp well in advance of the start date to determine if the staff can support your child's dietary needs. If you're concerned that the camp won't consistently provide gluten-free meals and snacks, provide the food yourself. One suggestion is to fill a large cooler and a suitcase with all of the food your child will need for a stay at overnight camp. Ask if a cafeteria staff member can be the point person for preparing your child's meals with this food. Or, if your child is able and willing, find out if he or she can help prepare the meals.

Don't hold your child back Encourage your child to take part in all activities that other kids do. It's better for them emotionally and socially. Just follow the extra precautions outlined above.

KEEPING YOUR TEENAGER ON TRACK The balancing act of staying gluten-free while trying to fit in can be particularly tough for teenagers. The teen years are a time of major changes in emotional, physical and intellectual development. As your child enters adolescence, you'll likely notice a strong desire to seek independence and question authority — or even rebel against it. Risk-taking also may seem more appealing. At the same time, friendships and other peer groups take on greater weight and influence. The desire to fit in and avoid standing out becomes very powerful. Along with these changes may come changing attitudes toward the gluten-free lifestyle.

Research shows that teenagers are more likely than their younger counterparts to knowingly cheat on a gluten-free diet. What's important to keep in mind is that the cheating may have little to do with the food itself. More often than not, a teenager who purposely eats food that contains gluten is attempting to avoid the perceived embarrassment of being different around friends. For that reason, the cheating tends to occur in social situations rather than at home.

Even if your child has stuck to a gluten-free diet up until now, be prepared for the possibility of a bumpier road through the teen years. With guidance and support, your child will move past this phase and gain the maturity to success-fully and independently manage the gluten-free diet for years to come.

Here are some ways you can help your teenager stay on track:

- **Don't stop teaching.** Teens who fully understand that the gluten-free diet is a long-term investment in their health are more likely to avoid cheating. On the other hand, if your teenager believes that a little pizza now and then won't hurt, he or she is more likely to eat it.

- **Nurture acceptance.** Teenagers who have come to terms with their condition are less likely to eat foods containing gluten.

- **Keep the lines of communication open.** Maintain a supportive attitude and encourage your teenager to be honest about his or her food struggles.

If cheating is an issue, ask about the reasons behind the cheating and help your teenager to problem-solve.

⚜ **Encourage openness with peers.** The more open your teenager is about his or her condition, the less of an issue it will be in social situations.

⚜ **Stress the value of supportive friends.** Teens who feel accepted and supported by their peers are more likely to stick to the gluten-free diet. If your teenager is struggling with negative or critical attitudes among some friends, let him or her know it's OK to avoid overly judgmental people.

⚜ **Help your teen plan ahead.** Teenagers may not be known for having great foresight, but this is exactly the skill they need to successfully maintain a gluten-free diet. The more your teen can anticipate food-related challenges in social situations, the easier it will be to work out viable solutions in advance.

Maneuvering the school scene

Many parents worry about how their children will handle the challenges of a gluten-free diet at school. With some extra planning and effort, you can ensure that your child has a safe and positive educational experience.

PREPARING YOUR CHILD FOR SCHOOL Whether your child is entering elementary school, middle school or high school, you can prepare him or her by offering practical guidance. The more your child can anticipate challenges — and be armed with solutions — the easier it will be to stay on target. Help your child navigate potential pitfalls at school with these suggestions:

⚜ **Be a self-advocate.** Coach your child on how to speak up about his or her gluten-free needs with school staff. Let him or her know it's OK to turn food down or ask for a gluten-free alternative.

⚜ **Avoid trading food.** Explain that trading food at lunch or snack time isn't safe, even if other classmates are doing it.

⚜ **If unsure, don't eat it.** If your child is offered food that isn't clearly labeled, he or she should know that's it's best not to eat it.

⚜ **Alert a teacher.** If your child accidently eats gluten or is experiencing symptoms, encourage your child to inform the teacher. The more your

Some schools voluntarily work with parents to create a safe environment for children with special dietary needs. Other school systems require specific documentation to meet those needs. Depending on the school your child attends, you may want to consider establishing a 504 plan. This formal document lays out the accommodations needed for your child to be safe and successful in school.

The 504 plan comes from Section 504 of the Rehabilitation Act of 1973, a federal law that prohibits discrimination on the basis of physical or mental disability. Programs that receive federal funding, including public school districts, are subject to this law and must consider petitions for 504 plans.

It's important to note that having celiac disease doesn't automatically qualify your child for services under a 504 plan. According to the National Foundation for Celiac Awareness (NFCA), your child's medical condition must cause a significant limitation to his or her ability to learn. If you choose to pursue a 504 plan, you'll be required to make an individualized argument for why your child should qualify and why lack of accommodation would be harmful to his or her education.

Each child's 504 plan is different. Some outline a few general accommodations, while others are quite specific. If you feel that a 504 plan would benefit your child, the NFCA and other celiac disease advocacy groups provide helpful information and sample documentation for parents wishing to pursue this option.

child's teachers are aware of his or her health, the more informed you'll be and it may give you some peace of mind.

* **Know which cafeteria foods are gluten-free.** The majority of children on a gluten-free diet bring their own lunches to school, but your child may want to buy food from the lunch line now and then. This may especially be the case once your child reaches middle school and seeks greater independence. With your child, figure out which foods are safe to eat and which should be avoided. Coach him or her on how to approach lunchroom staff if he or she has questions.

HELPING YOUR CHILD'S SCHOOL In addition to preparing your child for school, you want to prepare the school for your child. Meet with school staff and make them aware of your child's condition, the importance of a gluten-free diet, and how gluten affects your child's short- and long-term health. Here are some suggestions for educating key personnel and establishing a good relationship with staff.

Meet before school starts Set up a meeting with your child's teachers, school nurse, food services staff and others you feel should be included. You may ask to set up one meeting that includes everyone, or you may prefer to have individual meetings.

Create an informational packet Put together clear, concise and well-organized information about your child's condition. Be sure to include lists of foods that are and are not gluten-free. You may want to get a letter from your child's doctor confirming your child's medical condition and his or her dietary needs. Online support groups such as the Celiac Sprue Association and the National Foundation for Celiac Awareness (see pages 274 and 275) offer sample letters for parents to give to teachers, as well as other useful information to provide to your child's school.

Investigate school menus Most likely, your child will be bringing a packed lunch to school, but he or she may wish to occasionally purchase lunch. Find out if the school cafeteria offers any gluten-free meals or food items.

Supply the teacher with snacks Throughout the year, there are likely to be classroom celebrations or events that involve food. Make sure your child's teacher can offer your child a gluten-free snack when the rest of the class is enjoying a snack or treat.

Be alerted to birthdays If possible, find out when your child's classmates will be celebrating their birthdays at school. Or ask your child's teacher to alert you of upcoming birthday celebrations. If food will be involved, plan ahead so that your child will have a similar gluten-free treat.

Establish bathroom privileges Your child's condition may require an increased need to use the bathroom. Make sure teachers understand your child's bathroom needs.

Volunteer at school If possible, consider chaperoning field trips, helping out at lunchtime or being the homeroom parent. You may also choose to help lead after-school activities such as scout meetings. That way, you can observe what your son or daughter is eating without intruding.

Plan ahead for art projects Preschoolers and young children have a tendency to put their hands in their mouths. For that reason, they should avoid touching art supplies that contain gluten. Let teachers know that your child should avoid art projects that use gluten-containing supplies such as paste or papier-mache. Offer to make and donate gluten-free modeling clay for your child's classroom.

Be patient and positive Your attitude will set the stage for your relationship with your child's school. As you advocate for your child, maintain a polite and cooperative tone. Know that mistakes will likely be made as the school continues to learn about your child's needs. Address those mistakes head-on, but do so in a courteous way. School staff will be more likely to work with you if you show them respect and an appreciation for their efforts.

Heading off to college

If you're like most parents, the thought of your child entering college is both exciting and daunting. College represents a new level of independence for young adults — and a new set of challenges. Your worry may be compounded if your child needs to follow a gluten-free diet. Rest assured that with some extra diligence on your part and your child's, these challenges can be overcome.

As you research or visit prospective colleges, find out if they're set up to support students who need to eat gluten-free. If not, investigate whether they can adjust to accommodate your child. Larger universities may be more likely to have a system in place since they tend to have a larger number of students on special diets. You may also want to read the reviews on specific websites that allow students and parents to rate gluten-free options at various colleges and universities. Either way, don't let a gluten disorder prevent your child from attending the college of his or her choice.

While you research colleges, help your child prepare for greater independence and responsibility away from home. Ideally, you've been doing that all along by giving your child increasing control over his or her diet. Make sure your child knows how to read food labels, buy gluten-free groceries and prepare a variety of healthy gluten-free snacks and meals. Help your child anticipate problems that may arise, and make sure he or she knows how to respond. Once your child has decided on a school, he or she can follow these tips to make the transition to college a smoother one:

Contact food services Your child should speak with the person on campus that handles food allergies. This may be the food services director, head chef or a dietitian. Encourage your child to ask lots of questions. For example, how

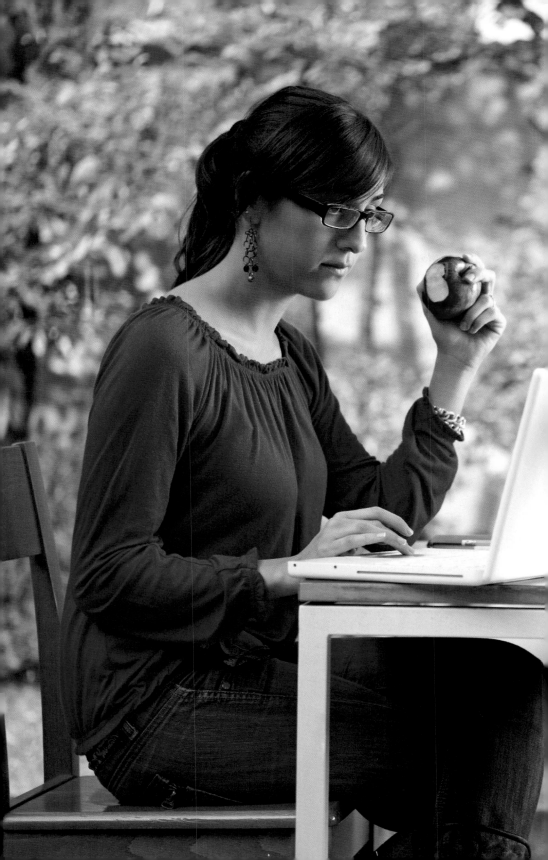

is food prepared and how is cross-contamination avoided? Are gluten-free foods labeled on the menu? Can the school provide your child with a complete list of food items and their ingredients? As much as possible, encourage your child's involvement in this process.

Become friendly with dining hall staff Your child should be prepared to politely advocate for him- or herself with the people preparing dining hall meals. Encourage your child to speak up if he or she has questions or concerns about unknown ingredients and food preparation.

Register with the office that oversees students with disabilities Doing so can help protect his or her right to a safe environment on campus and may allow for certain accommodations. Your child will likely need a letter from his or her doctor and will have to fill out some forms.

Locate a good grocery store nearby If there isn't one, figure out ways to purchase gluten-free food online. Having a stash of gluten-free foods and snacks will come in handy when the dining hall isn't an option.

Request a dorm with a kitchen That way, your child can prepare gluten-free meals and snacks when needed. Some larger schools may even offer dorms with kitchens reserved specifically for students on special diets.

Bring small appliances Ask what appliances are allowed in dorm rooms. Having access to a microwave, small refrigerator, and toaster can make eating gluten-free a lot easier.

Communicate with roommates Your child will need to educate roommates about his or her condition and agree on a plan to avoid cross-contamination in the dorm room.

Leading the way

Whatever stage of life your child is in, your support and guidance will be invaluable. Your ongoing efforts to teach coping skills and share knowledge with your child will help him or her learn from mistakes and master the gluten-free lifestyle. By keeping the lines of communication open and working together to resolve problems, your child can thrive at home, school and everywhere in between.

Moving forward

Having celiac disease or another gluten- or wheat-related disorder means making a significant change in what you eat. Change often isn't easy, but it's helpful to know that your actions will bring big rewards. As your body begins to heal from years of food-related illness, you may find that you feel healthier than you have in a long time.

As you've likely learned — from personal experience and from reading this book — managing a gluten-free diet is a learning process. In the beginning, the changes to your diet and to your routines can be demanding, but living with your condition gets easier with time. Your goal is to master your new diet so that it no longer masters you. It's a goal you can, and will, achieve.

As you move forward, stay positive, take good care of yourself, and enjoy the journey to a healthier you.

Your life isn't defined by your illness

Chances are, your illness has affected not only what you put in your mouth but, to some extent, how you function and live your life. You've likely changed the way you shop for food, what you cook, where you eat out, how you travel and the way you prepare for social gatherings. For these reasons, your condition has affected not just you but your family and others close to you.

Your need to avoid gluten may be a fact of life, but it doesn't need to define your life. Having a gluten disorder isn't a prison sentence. Instead, think of it as an opportunity to enjoy a healthier lifestyle. You may discover that you're more resilient and adaptable than you ever thought you could be. You may even find that your new lifestyle has opened you up to unexpected pleasures.

With practice, patience and some planning, you'll find that daily life can feel normal again.

Caring for your whole self

Living well without gluten is more than just watching what you eat. As you deal with the ups and downs of a gluten-free diet, keep tabs on your physical, mental and emotional well-being.

GET ENOUGH SLEEP Sleep is important. Most people seem to need about eight hours of sleep a night to feel rested. But that varies from person to person. If you feel alert and function well during the day and don't feel like sleeping when you sit down and relax, you're probably getting enough sleep.

Many people who begin a gluten-free diet find they have more energy, and they feel less fatigued. This is likely because they're feeling better, they're eating healthier, and their bodies are getting nutrients they were lacking. Don't be surprised if you find that you need less sleep than before you changed your diet, or that you're sleeping better now that your body is healing.

EXERCISE Exercising regularly can help you cope more effectively with all of the challenges of life. Along with improving your mood, exercise provides many other benefits. It can give you more energy, help you lose weight, help keep your bones strong, help you sleep better, and give you a greater sense of confidence and self-worth.

Many people find that as their health improves they have more stamina and energy. With this newfound energy, it's easier to be physically active and get regular exercise.

Adding more activity to your life needn't be a chore. Find something you like to do. It might be cycling, swimming, playing tennis or ballroom dancing. Exercises such as yoga and Zumba are beneficial too, as are strengthening exercises such as resistance training and weightlifting. An easy way to incorporate more physical activity into your life is to walk more. Walking is a great exercise that virtually anyone can do.

If you haven't exercised much and you want to take part in a more vigorous exercise program or you have severe osteoporosis, talk with your doctor before you begin. Otherwise, put on a pair of tennis shoes and take a walk!

PRACTICE RELAXATION Everyone experiences stress, but the challenges of a chronic illness can increase your level of stress. Relaxation techniques can help you release tension and improve your health and quality of life. Relaxation means more than occasional time to rest or enjoying a favorite hobby. It involves taking a break from your daily tasks and responsibilities and eliminating built-up tension from your body.

Common relaxation techniques include meditation, relaxed breathing, muscle relaxation and visualization. Massage, prayer, and listening to soothing music or nature sounds also can help you relax and gain a greater sense of calm. Try out different forms of relaxation to see which ones work best for you. With practice, these techniques will become automatic.

Learning to relax and refuel provides many benefits. In addition to improving your mood, when you're relaxed you have a better sense of control over your health and you're better equipped to deal with life's challenges. This is important when making major changes to your diet.

BE MINDFUL To be mindful means to focus — intentionally and with purpose — on what's going on with you right now. When you're mindful, you're present in the moment. You accept whatever is happening. It is what it is. You don't judge or label things as good or bad.

One of the nice things about being mindful is that you can do it anytime, anywhere. For example, if you go for a walk, focus on what you're seeing, hearing and smelling. Is the floor smooth or rough? What sounds do you hear? If you're trying a new food, it can help you keep an open mind when exploring its tastes and textures.

Incorporating mindfulness into your life can help you relax and react less to stress. It can also help you manage negative thoughts, become a better problem solver, and develop more gratitude for the good things and people in your life.

Gaining perspective

The information in this book can help you more easily adapt to a gluten-free diet. Keep in mind that change takes time and practice. Expect a few setbacks as you get used to your new diet, but know that with time you will become an expert at all things gluten. As you make your way on the path to better health, living gluten-free will feel less like a burden. Your condition is only a piece of your life, not the whole of it.

RYAN'S STORY

My experience with celiac disease is both typical and not so typical. Although I didn't realize it at the time, I'd been suffering from common symptoms like digestive problems and fatigue for around 10 years. I thought they were due to stress and poor eating habits. I didn't know that I was slowly poisoning my body with gluten.

One day at work, my body kind of shut down. I started to hear a loud ringing in my ears and lost hearing in my left ear. I also lost all sense of balance, and my brain felt like it was jiggling in my head. The symptoms hit me like a freight train.

My doctor had concerns about the hearing loss and referred me to an ear, nose and throat doctor. That doctor then referred me to a neurologist, but no neurological tests could explain my symptoms. I finally got tested for celiac disease, and that's how I received my diagnosis. It was a huge relief. Finally, there might be a reason for my symptoms and — even better — a treatment. I went gluten-free and I haven't looked back since.

Right away, my wife and I went through our kitchen and identified foods I couldn't eat. After I cut out all gluten from my diet, I started to feel better pretty quickly. My energy level improved and so did my digestive problems. After about six weeks, my neurological symptoms also started to get better. Even so, the symptoms would sometimes flare up for what seemed like no reason. My wife and I couldn't figure out what was wrong, but after doing some research we realized I might be getting some contamination right in my own kitchen. We cleaned our cooking utensils thoroughly, bought some new kitchen supplies just for me, and cleared out one cupboard for my gluten-free food. I also learned that I needed to read food labels very carefully.

Early on, my wife and three young children would share gluten-free meals with me. They still ate foods containing gluten at home, but usually not at family meals. Just recently, our family decided to make our household entirely gluten-free. We've discovered that it's easier to avoid cross-contamination that way. I've been surprised by how well my children have adapted to the change. They don't seem to mind eating gluten-free waffles, chips and other foods.

My friends have been supportive, too. At first I had to coach them on my condition and how it affects what I'm able to eat. Over time, they've adapted their cooking when I come over.

It's been a year since my diagnosis, and I feel healthier than I have in many years. I don't miss my old diet, except for not being able to drink a greater variety of domestic and imported beers. But that doesn't feel like much of a sacrifice or burden. The gluten-free diet has given me my health back! That's worth all the beer, bread and pasta in the world.

ADDITIONAL RESOURCES

Academy of Nutrition and Dietetics
120 S. Riverside Plaza, Suite 2000
Chicago, IL 60606-6995
800-877-1600
www.eatright.org

American Celiac Disease Alliance
2504 Duxbury Place
Alexandria, VA 22308
703-622-3331
http://americanceliac.org

Asthma and Allergy Foundation of America
8201 Corporate Drive, Suite 1000
Landover, MD 20785
800-727-8462
www.aafa.org

Canadian Celiac Association
5025 Orbitor Drive
Building 1, Suite 400
Mississauga, ON L4W 4Y5
Canada
800-363-7296
www.celiac.ca

Celiac Disease Foundation
20350 Ventura Blvd., Suite 240
Woodland Hills, CA 91364
818-716-1513
http://celiac.org

Celiac Sprue Association
see Celiac Support Association

Celiac Support Association
P.O. Box 31700
1941 S. 42nd St., Suite 522
Omaha, NE 68105

877-272-4272
www.csaceliacs.info

Cel-Kids Network
see Celiac Support Association

FARE (Food Allergy Research & Education)
7925 Jones Branch Drive, Suite 1100
McLean, VA 22102
800-929-4040
www.foodallergy.org

Gluten-Free Certification Organization
see Gluten Intolerance Group

Gluten Intolerance Group
31212 124th Ave. SE
Auburn, WA 98092
253-833-6655
www.gluten.net

Mayo Clinic
www.MayoClinic.org

National Digestive Diseases Information Clearinghouse
2 Information Way
Bethesda, MD 20892-3570
800-891-5389
http://digestive.niddk.nih.gov

National Foundation for Celiac Awareness
P.O. Box 544
124 S. Maple St.
Ambler, PA 19002-0544
215-325-1306
www.celiaccentral.org

R.O.C.K. (Raising Our Celiac Kids)
National Celiac Disease Support Group
www.celiac.com

INDEX

HLA-DQ2/HLA-DQ8 genes, 70–72
human leukocyte antigen (HLA) genes,
    22–25, 70–72, 74
"hygiene hypothesis," 30

I

IBS (irritable bowel syndrome), 109
ileum, 20, 22
immunoglobulin E (IgE), 139
incorrect diagnosis, 79, 105, 108
infertility, 45
inflammatory bowel disease, 119
ingredients, food labels, 184
insurance coverage, 66
international travel, 240, 242
intestinal lining, 22, 92
iron, 96, 150
irritable bowel syndrome (IBS), 109
isolation, feelings of, 249–250

J

Jewish traditions, 255
joint problems, 44–45

K

kitchen
    appliances, contaminated, 202–203
    cleaning, 201–202
    organization, 227
    restocking, 197–213
    utensils, contaminated, 202–203

L

labels. See food labels; gluten-free labels
lactose, 132
lactose intolerance
    celiac disease and, 36, 94, 109
    gluten-free diet and, 170
    test, 94
life
    full, enjoying, 255
    moving forward in, 270–272
    not defined by illness, 270–271
    whole self-care, 271–272
living with celiac disease
    coming to terms with, 80–89
    control and, 83–84
    normal feelings, 81–83
    options, 84
    perspective, 89
    seeking out dietitian and, 84–86
    support, finding, 86–89

logos, certification, 186–188
lunch
    on gluten-free diet, 170
    simple suggestions, 172

M

mac and cheese, 220
male concerns, 45–46
malnutrition, 133
malt, 191
management, celiac disease
    in children, 96
    expectations, 91–95
    follow-up visits, 97–99
    nutrients, 96–97
    overview of, 90–91
    symptoms, 91–92
    weight, 92
meal planning
    family and, 217
    grocery shopping and, 210
    leftovers and, 217
    plan creation, 85
    schedule and, 216
    visual guide, 167
    weekly, 215–217
meal replacement beverages, 207
meals, simple ideas, 172–173
meats
    best gluten-free options, 163–164
    grocery shopping for, 208
medications
    gluten in, 194–195
    wheat allergy, 143
menstruation, abnormal, 45
mesquite four, 229
microscopic colitis, 28, 110
millet, 178
millet flour, 229
minerals, 96, 148–150, 168
mobile apps, 193
multivitamins, 90, 195
myths, celiac disease, 51–53

N

National Digestive Diseases Information
    Clearinghouse, 275
National Foundation for Celiac
    Awareness, 275
nocebo effect, 129
non-celiac gluten sensitivity (NCGS)
    debate, 125

MAYO CLINIC

Housecall

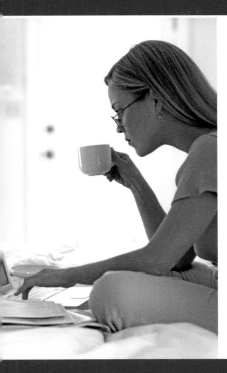

What our readers are saying ...

*"I depend on **Mayo Clinic Housecall** more than any other medical info that shows up on my computer. Thank you so very much."*

"Excellent newsletter. I always find something interesting to read and learn something new."

*"**Housecall** is a must read – keep up the good work!"*

*"I love **Housecall**. It is one of the most useful, trusted and beneficial things that come from the Internet."*

Get the latest health information direct from Mayo Clinic ... Sign up today, it's FREE!

Mayo Clinic Housecall is a FREE weekly e-newsletter that offers the latest health information from the experts at Mayo Clinic. Stay up to date on topics that are current, interesting, and most of all important to your health and the health of your family.

What you get
- Weekly top story
- Additional healthy highlights
- Answers from the experts
- Quick access to trusted health tools
- Featured blogs
- Health tip of the week
- Special offers

Don't wait ... Join today!
MayoClinic.com/Housecall/Register

We're committed to helping you enjoy better health and get the most out of life every day. We hope you decide to become part of the Mayo Clinic family, where you can always count on receiving an interesting mix of health information from a trusted source.

More great Mayo Clinic publications

Visit **www.store.MayoClinic.com** for reliable Mayo Clinic publications to help with your top health interests.

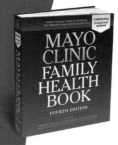

Mayo Clinic Family Health Book
Completely revised and updated Fourth Edition
It's your owner's manual for the human body.

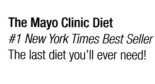

Mayo Clinic on Digestive Health
Learn how to identify and treat digestive problems before they become difficult to manage.

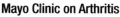

The Mayo Clinic Diet
#1 New York Times Best Seller
The last diet you'll ever need!

Mayo Clinic on Arthritis
Better medications, improved treatments and self-care tips to lead a more active, comfortable life.

Many more popular titles to choose from ...

» Mayo Clinic on Healthy Aging

» Mayo Clinic on Alzheimer's Disease

» The Mayo Clinic Breast Cancer Book

» Mayo Clinic Essential Diabetes Book

» The Mayo Clinic Diabetes Diet

» The Mayo Clinic Diabetes Diet Journal

» Mayo Clinic Healthy Heart for Life

» Mayo Clinic Fitness for EveryBody

» Fix-It And Enjoy-It Healthy Cookbook

» Mayo Clinic Guide to Your Baby's First Year

» Mayo Clinic Guide to a Healthy Pregnancy

» Mayo Clinic on Better Hearing and Balance

» Mayo Clinic 5 Steps to Controlling High Blood Pressure

» Mayo Clinic Book of Home Remedies

» Mayo Clinic on Managing Incontinence

» The Mayo Clinic Kids' Cookbook

» The New Mayo Clinic Cookbook

» The Mayo Clinic Diet Journal

» Mayo Clinic Guide to Preventing and Treating Osteoporosis

» Mayo Clinic Essential Guide to Prostate Health

» Mayo Clinic Guide to Better Vision

Learn more at
www.store.MayoClinic.com